THE COMPLETE GUIDE TO

SHAPING UP

A STRUCTURED COURSE
IN WEIGHT TRAINING
FOR MEN AND WOMEN

KYLE RODERICK

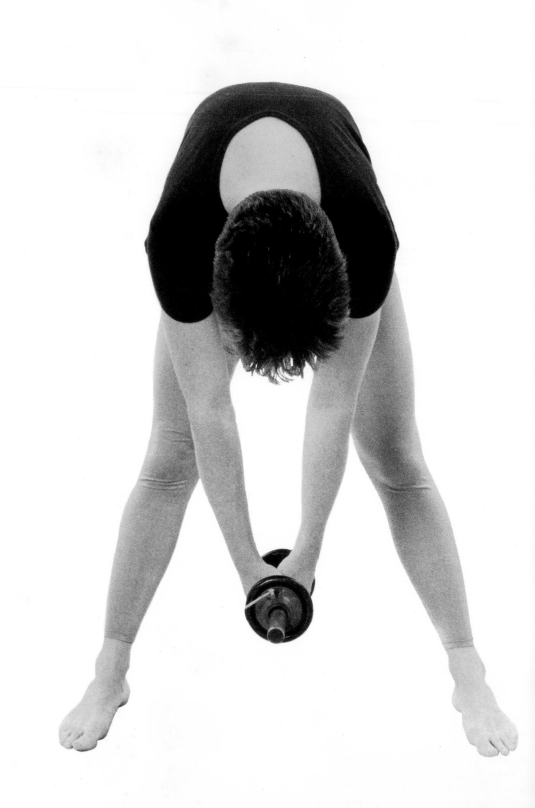

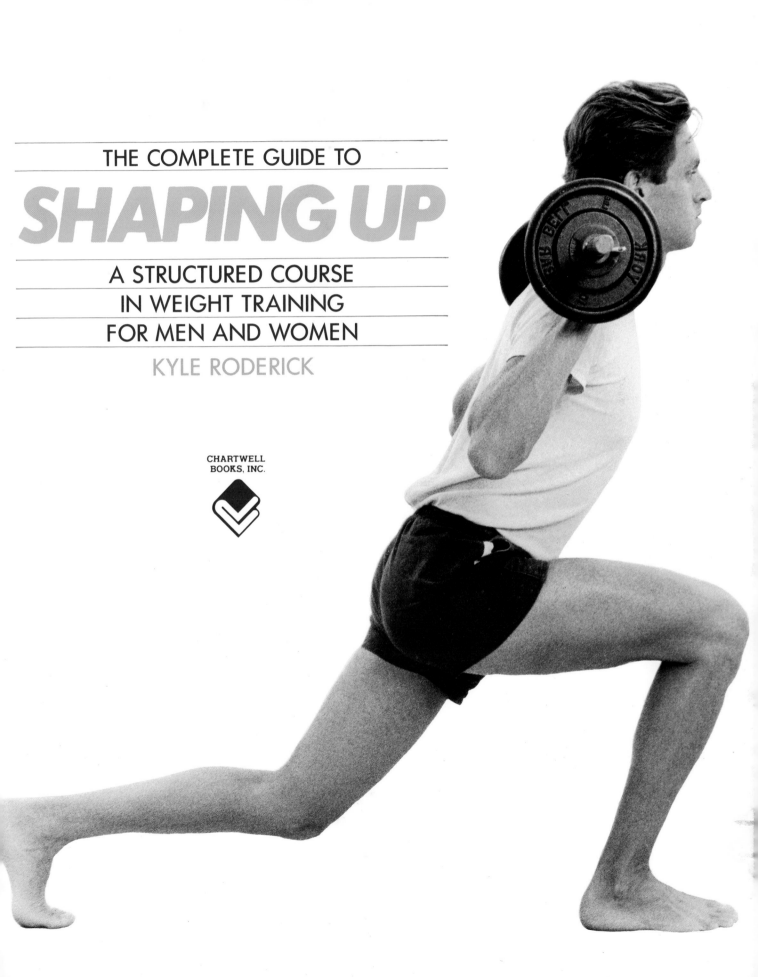

THE COMPLETE GUIDE TO
SHAPING UP

A STRUCTURED COURSE
IN WEIGHT TRAINING
FOR MEN AND WOMEN

KYLE RODERICK

CHARTWELL
BOOKS, INC.

A QUINTET BOOK

Published by Chartwell Books Inc.,
A Division of Book Sales Inc.,
110 Enterprise Avenue,
Secaucus, New Jersey 07094

ISBN 0-89009-854-9

This book was designed and produced by
Quintet Publishing Limited
6 Blundell Street, London N7

Art design by Mixed Media
Photographer Cyndy Warwick
Editor Stephen Paul

Typeset in Great Britain by
Q.V. Typesetting Limited, London
Colour origination in Hong Kong by
Hong Kong Graphic Arts Company Limited, Hong Kong
Printed in Hong Kong by Leefung-Asco
Printers Limited

Contents

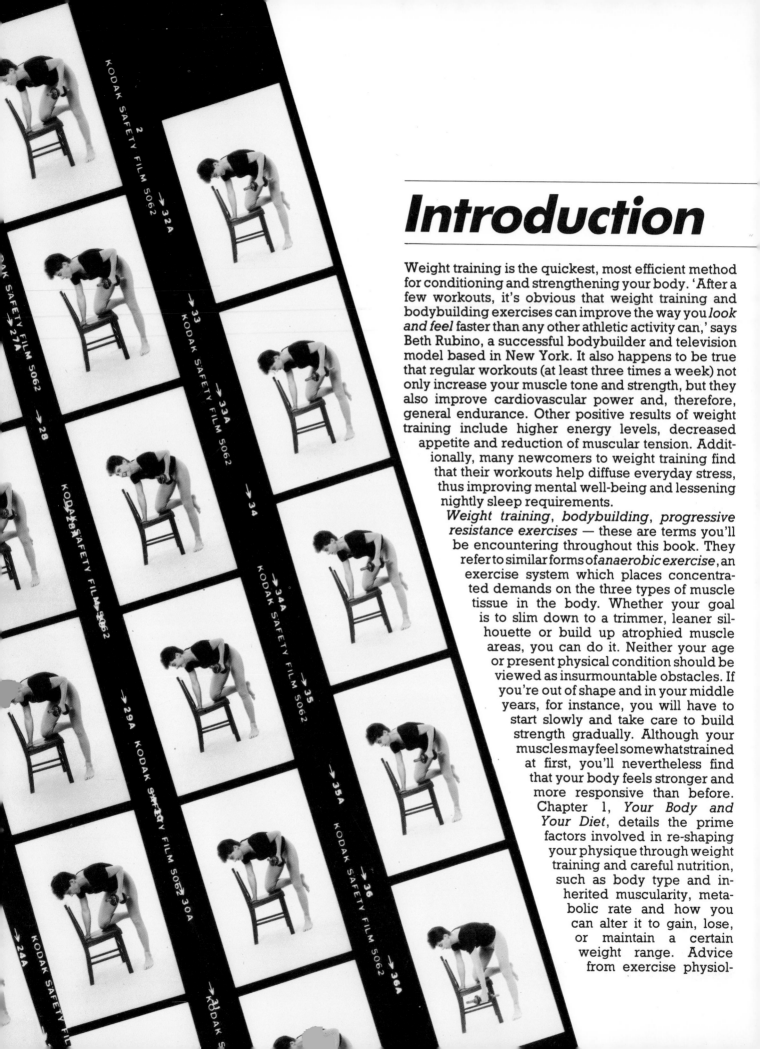

Introduction

Weight training is the quickest, most efficient method for conditioning and strengthening your body. 'After a few workouts, it's obvious that weight training and bodybuilding exercises can improve the way you *look and feel* faster than any other athletic activity can,' says Beth Rubino, a successful bodybuilder and television model based in New York. It also happens to be true that regular workouts (at least three times a week) not only increase your muscle tone and strength, but they also improve cardiovascular power and, therefore, general endurance. Other positive results of weight training include higher energy levels, decreased appetite and reduction of muscular tension. Additionally, many newcomers to weight training find that their workouts help diffuse everyday stress, thus improving mental well-being and lessening nightly sleep requirements.

Weight training, *bodybuilding*, *progressive resistance exercises* — these are terms you'll be encountering throughout this book. They refer to similar forms of *anaerobic exercise*, an exercise system which places concentrated demands on the three types of muscle tissue in the body. Whether your goal is to slim down to a trimmer, leaner silhouette or build up atrophied muscle areas, you can do it. Neither your age or present physical condition should be viewed as insurmountable obstacles. If you're out of shape and in your middle years, for instance, you will have to start slowly and take care to build strength gradually. Although your muscles may feel somewhat strained at first, you'll nevertheless find that your body feels stronger and more responsive than before. Chapter 1, *Your Body and Your Diet*, details the prime factors involved in re-shaping your physique through weight training and careful nutrition, such as body type and inherited muscularity, metabolic rate and how you can alter it to gain, lose, or maintain a certain weight range. Advice from exercise physiologists and nutritionists guides you toward eating for more energy and muscle, and checklists for pinpointing the quality of your diet are also included. The four basic food groups and nutrients are explained so that you can gain an awareness of how to balance your diet while still satisfying your tastes. Menu plans for three meals a day are provided to get you started on healthier eating habits. There's even a caloric breakdown of hundreds of nutritious foods, courtesy of a world class bodybuilder, Lydia Cheng.

And, in case you're curious about how best to supplement your meals, there's a primer on the essential properties of major vitamins and minerals, and a list of what foods they can be obtained from.

Chapter 2, *Getting Your Body In Gear*, concerns itself mainly with everything you need to know about muscle. Beginning with a discussion of the inherent differences between men's and women's physiques, descriptions of muscle-to-body fat ratios, endurance levels and other vital specifics, the chapter enables you to visualize how *your* body will respond to weight training and other forms of exercise. Illustrations of the major muscles and muscle groups demonstrate the relationships of muscle tissue in the body, and a checklist for appraising your muscle tone and strength is supplied so that you can identify 'trouble spots' where you may need to do extra work when you begin weight training in earnest. The results of this fitness checklist also serve to determine which workout plan you should start with: the exercises are divided into beginning, intermediate and advanced workouts.

Because many people who train with weights want to develop strength — but not massive muscles — a section detailing the benefits of *aerobic* exercise is also included. You can complement your weight training with aerobic sports that burn up lots of calories and body weight, and thus maintain your muscularity at a desirable level. The chapter concludes with advice from bodybuilders on how to avoid and/or treat injuries.

Chapter 3, *The Beginning Workout Plan*, is a comprehensive program designed especially for the beginner. The exercises from Chapter 2's fitness level checklist can be done as warm-ups for this and the other workouts in the book. *The Beginning Workout Plan* places special emphasis on completing the exercises with proper breathing, movement and concentration. Beginners needn't worry about the amount of weight they are (or aren't) lifting at first. In order to

lift heavier weights and build strength, one first has to develop *proper* form and some basic muscle tone.

The majority of the exercises in this section can be done anywhere, anytime — at the office, at home, or, if you happen to move around a lot, you can even do them in your hotel room. Furniture, books and hand weights are the only equipment you need. Thus, the investment in a sleeker, stronger body is minimal. All you really have to invest in is time: at least three times a week.

Chapter 4's *Intermediate Workout Plan* contains some variations on exercises in the preceding chapter, but there are also some exercises that are best done in a gym, using professional equipment. You should progress to this *Intermediate* level *only* after you can complete the *Beginning Workout* with minimal exertion. Some people do progress faster than others, however, so you may be ready to move on to these exercises after only a month of beginning weight training. Women, especially, should not be discouraged by slow progress in either the *Beginning* or *Intermediate* sections. Exercise physiologists have concluded that women's physical endurance is actually superior to men's, so keep this in mind as you try to reach those long-term fitness goals.

Chapter 5, *The Advanced Workout Plan*, is mainly composed of exercises to be done in a weight training gym. These exercises involve relatively heavy weights and multiple repetitions. Because they are rather strenuous, it is important to complete each movement with due care and attention. Accidental injury is always a possibility, no matter how strong you may feel you are.

Chapter 6, *Keeping Your Shape*, covers a wide spectrum of bodybuilding/weight training topics: information that you need to know regarding maintaining your shape; whether or not to work out when ill; and the relative merits of different kinds of equipment, from free weights to machines, slant boards and incline benches. Bodybuilders and trainers comment on these topics, so the enthusiastic beginner can gain an insider's knowledge of weight training and how this rapidly developing sport can improve physical and mental well-being.

The Complete Guide to Shaping-Up is the answer to every body's needs. All it takes is patience and a few weeks of working out and you will soon see the improvements in your physique, and feel the increased energy and responsiveness of both mind and body.

Chapter 1

Evaluating your body and your diet

Getting into peak physical condition is impossible without first understanding what approximate body type you are, what your present level of fitness is and how healthy your eating habits are. Before you start any exercise program, it's a good idea to have a complete medical check-up. Take note of your blood pressure and your resting pulse rate. Your doctor should be able to advise you of what's normal for your age, sex and degree of activity.

Many people still mistakenly believe that if they can only exercise enough, then they'll be in 'good health'. They're right, up to a point, but careful nutrition coupled with regular exercise is really the only way to get yourself in optimum shape. Accordingly, much of this chapter focuses on teaching you how to analyze your physical and dietary strengths and weaknesses. Topics such as body composition and the specific properties of different nutrients are detailed so that you gain a holistic awareness of how to fuel and work your body with maximum efficiency. After all, the food you eat affects your physical performance, and vice versa.

To get an initial idea of your physical condition, take off your clothes and study your body in a full-length mirror. Starting at your shoulders, note the shape and muscle tone of your individual body parts. Look at your arms, chest, waistline, hips, upper legs and calves. How does your posture rate? Is your body harmoniously proportioned? Are there any areas where you are obviously out of shape, such as the waist, stomach, lower back, thighs, or upper arms? One way to tell if you are carrying too much fat is to do the skinfold test. Start by pinching some of your skin between your thumb and forefinger. The best areas for this are the triceps (back of the upper arm), the side of the waist and the top of the thigh. If you can pinch more than half an inch of skin, this means that you have excess body fat, and you need to exercise and/or lose weight.

The main thing to remember when confronting parts of your body that are out of shape is not to be discouraged! You can easily change for the better. This demands a daily commitment, however, and you must realize that it may take several months to achieve the results you want. The following chapters are geared towards helping you plan a diet, exercise and weight training program that will help you to improve all aspects of your physique.

Another vital point you must understand before you start exercising with weights to re-shape your body is your *approximate physical type*. This is determined by two decisive elements: body type and body composition. Body type refers to your inherited genetic structure, and body composition describes the ratio of muscle to fat in your body weight. (Women's bodies contain approximately 25 per cent more fat cells than men's, thus, women have fewer muscle cells than men.)

Although body composition can be altered by careful diet and exercise, your body type is essentially fixed for life. That is to say, if you are born with large bones and a muscular build, your body will probably never look super-lean or slight. You can, however, re-shape and define your build by slimming down — or building muscle — through a balanced diet and exercise program.

Body types are divided into three categories:
Ectomorph: Long boned and thin, ectomorphs tend to gain weight with difficulty, and have relatively small muscle mass.
Mesomorph: This body type is muscular, strong and husky. Mesomorphs are usually medium to large boned.
Endomorph: With a tendency to gain weight easily, endomorphic bodies are relatively curvy and soft.

According to Dr Jairo Rodriguez, who is a New York chiropractor, clinical nutritionist and kinesiologist (kinesiology is the study of muscles and muscle movement), 'Each individual is a combination of the three categories. You will never find an individual who is a total ectomorph, for instance. More often than not people have mixed characteristics like a very lean upper body and a heavier, curvy lower body. Individuals with a high muscle mass in the upper body, with a very low fat, low muscle mass in the lower body are also quite common.'

Dr Rodriguez counsels that the most sensible way to begin a diet and weight training program is by having a medical professional evaluate your blood chemistry,

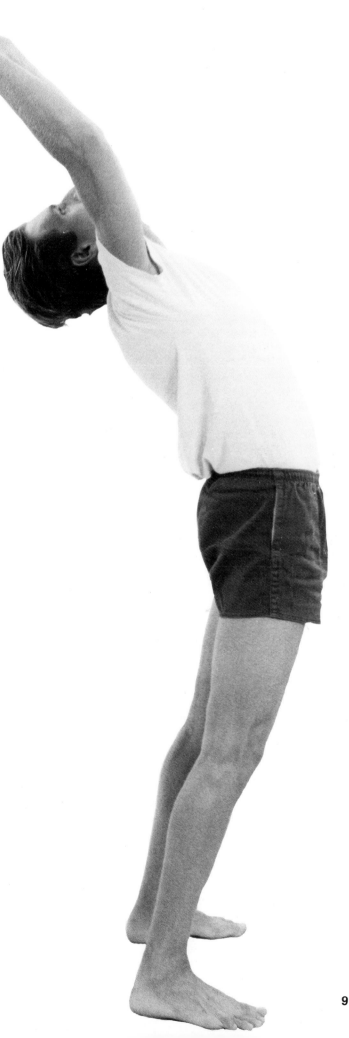

body fat percentage and bone size. This kind of thorough check-up will detect any bio-chemical imbalances that may exist, as well as indicate the type of excercise program that best suits your physique. For instance, some people's bodies require vigorous aerobic exercise (such as running or swimming) in addition to a weight training program in order to lose weight and build up atrophied muscles. Only a professional analysis of your physical make-up can pinpoint how *your body* works and what its needs are. Specific factors such as metabolic rate, bone size, natural muscularity and body fat percentages not only influence your ability to gain and lose weight, they also dictate the degree to which you can expect to build muscle mass and strength.

Depending on what body type you resemble, you may be interested in further details about how your physique will most likely respond to weight training. Ectomesomorphs, to begin with, usually have an efficient metabolic rate that rapidly burns up calories and stores a relatively low amount of fat. Although ectomesomorphs can build muscle through weight training and other programmed exercise, results can be difficult to achieve. Increased strength and muscle may take months of serious workouts.

The genetic endowment of mesomorphs predisposes them to developing strength, endurance and muscle well beyond the average. It's no accident that many champion athletes have classic mesomorphic bodies — tennis player Martina Navratilova, soccer star Pele and ballet dancer Mikhail Baryshnikov are just a few examples.

Endomorphs, because they carry more fat under their skin than other body types, often look less muscular than they truly are. Dieting is never easy for endomorphs, although building strength and muscle poses no challenge. If you happen to be an endomorph who wants to lose weight, your first priority should be devising a low fat, balanced diet that gives you enough energy for weight training and other forms of exercise. The following sections on diet and clinical nutrition are designed to tone, strengthen and re-shape *your particular* body type, for weight training cannot do it alone. Programmed exercise — plus diet — is the key.

The Quality of Your Diet

Although we spend significant amounts of time shopping for food, preparing it, and consuming meals, most of us know very little about food and how it can nourish or damage every cell in our bodies. Some basic, practical knowledge of nutrition is essential if you want to lose weight, live healthier and longer, and reap maximum benefits from your weight training program. Food does much more for you than simply provide energy to get through the day. To begin with, it can increase, or decrease, your mental concentration. More importantly, however, eating nutritious foods will ensure that your cells and tissues grow, maintain and repair themselves. Certain foods can also help regulate different internal body processes. A 'balanced diet' involves eating a variety of foods from the four basic food groups: milk and milk products; meats and other protein sources such as eggs, cheese, fish, dry beans and nuts; fruits and vegetables, and breads and cereals. Although the major nutrients of the four food groups are proteins, carbohydrates and fats, your body also requires nutrients such as water, fibre and air.

Carbohydrates

Carbohydrates fuel the world's population with most of its energy, for they are cheaper and easier to obtain and store than the prime protein sources. Found in sugar and starches, carbohydrates are compounded of carbon, hydrogen and oxygen. Starch is the main supplier of the carbohydrates that we eat, and since it is a complex sugar, the body has to break it down into simple sugars before it can be used as energy. If you're watching your weight, don't forget to take starch into account as part of your total sugar intake. Relatively high in calories, the main sources of starch are: rice, pasta, flour, potatoes, cereals and breads.

As for sugar, there are actually several different types of it. *Sucrose* is the substance that we usually refer to as sugar, and it is found in sugar beet and sugar cane. *Maltose* is made naturally from starch during the germination of grain, as well as in the production of malt liquors. *Lactose* (milk sugar) is present in animal and human milk, and is used to make butter and margarine. When the body breaks down complex sugars and starch, it produces its own sugar, called *glucose*. Glucose is the substance that carries fuel to your organs and muscles.

Sugar has absolutely no nutritional value. It is pure energy for the body. High in calorific content, sugar gives your system a quick lift, but lets you down soon afterwards. Refined (white) sugar, brown sugar, maple syrup, honey or molasses — they are equally debilitating to your health. Sugar is the major cause of tooth decay, and contributes to overweight, mood fluctuations, and irregularities in the body's blood sugar levels. In excess amounts, all sugars convert immediately to fat, so why not try satisfying your sweet tooth with fresh fruit instead. At least you'll be consuming fibre, vitamins and minerals instead of just empty calories. After all, fructose, the type of sugar found in fruits, vegetables and honey, is the sweetest sugar you can eat! Because the average person's sugar consumption is mainly through high fat foods like ice cream and baked goods, you will probably lose excess weight faster if you restrict your sugar intake exclusively to fruit and vegetable sources.

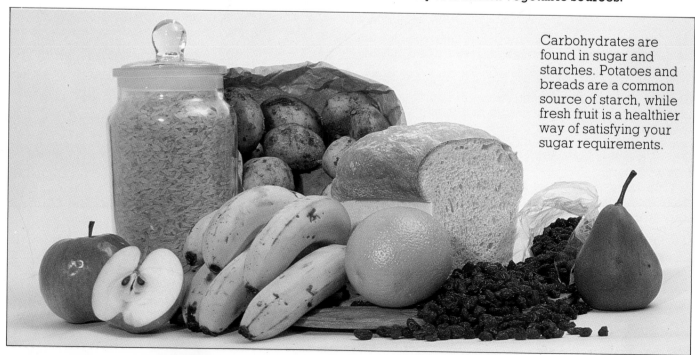

Carbohydrates are found in sugar and starches. Potatoes and breads are a common source of starch, while fresh fruit is a healthier way of satisfying your sugar requirements.

Protein

Apart from water, protein is the most common substance in the body cells, accounting for about 12 per cent of our body weight. It consists of hydrogen, carbon, nitrogen, and in some cases, phosphorus and sulphur. Protein also helps build and repair muscles, ligaments, nails and hair. It's also present in the red blood cells, the digestive enzymes and insulin. Protein contains an estimated 22 amino acids, of which 10 cannot be made by the body. After the digestive enzymes synthesize the protein from our food into 'constituent' amino acids, the body uses these to create its own protein. And, if we ingest more protein than our body needs, the excess is either burned up as energy or stored as body fat.

It is difficult to dictate a standard daily protein requirement. Age, sex, degree of activity and health history are all vital factors in determining your nutritional profile. Generally speaking, however, nutritionists recommend about 1¾ oz (50 grams) a day. High protein foods include: poultry, fish, milk, eggs, cheese and meat. Also, tofu (soybean curd), peas, beans, nuts, cereals and cereal products. Vegetarians should be advised that most plant proteins are often low in one essential amino acid. It's therefore a wise idea for them to plan meals that include the widest variety of plants available.

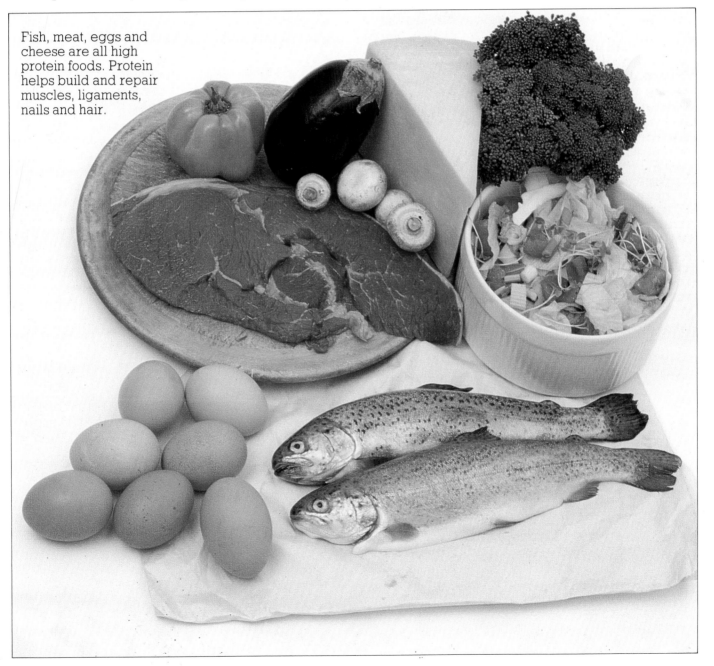

Fish, meat, eggs and cheese are all high protein foods. Protein helps build and repair muscles, ligaments, nails and hair.

Fats

Composed of carbon, hydrogen and oxygen, fats have an energy value that is twice the amount of protein or carbohydrates. All fats are thus high calorie foods, besides being a highly concentrated energy source. Fats also facilitate the transport of fat-soluble vitamins like A, D, E and K throughout the body. Additionally, linoleic acid, which is essential for healthy, elastic skin, can only be produced by fats. Because they are digested so slowly, fats work to prevent the feeling of hunger long after you've eaten a meal. Since they play such a vital role in the diet and have complex properties, a further explanation of fats is in order.

Different Types of Fats: How Do They Affect Your Body?

Fats are made up of fatty acids and glycerol. Each fatty acid is formed by chains of carbon atoms which have hydrogen atoms attached to them. Whenever each carbon atom has the maximum possible number of hydrogen atoms attached, it is known as *saturated* fat. The various patterns of carbon-hydrogen atoms produce *mono-unsaturated* and *polyunsaturated* fats. Saturated fat is found in all foods from animal sources, namely, meat and dairy products. Lard, suet, meat, poultry and fatty fish drippings — these are extremely high in saturated fats, and difficult for the body to break down and digest. Other foods loaded with saturated fat include: butter, hard cheeses, hard margarine, cream, full fat milk and coconut oil.

All saturated fats contain cholesterol, a fat-like substance which is formed naturally inside animal and human bodies. Too much cholesterol in the bloodstream causes a build-up of fatty deposits on the inside walls of the arteries, thus reducing their width and impeding the flow of blood to the heart. A condition like this can sometimes lead to a heart attack, so please

be advised that saturated fats are a serious risk factor contributing to the rise of high blood cholesterol and coronary heart disease. Close to 40 per cent of the calories we consume daily are supplied by fats, and the majority of these are saturated ones.

Because of the health risks just described, major medical clinics and researchers around the world recommend that you reduce the intake of saturated fats in your diet by a third. In any case, if you're committed to maintaining optimum health and controlling your weight, your eating habits can easily be re-structured and improved. Begin by keeping a journal of every meal, snack or 'taste' that you eat in a week. After seven days, calculate how much fat, saturated fats and cholesterol you normally consume. Then begin planning your meals to ensure that your daily intake has been reduced to the following specifications:

— ¼ less total fat consumption
— ⅓ less saturated fat consumption
— ½ less cholesterol consumption
— ⅓ MORE POLYUNSATURATED FAT.

You may well be curious about what *poly-unsaturated* means, and why these fats are indeed better for you than others. Polyunsaturated fats come mainly in foods from vegetable sources, such as margarine, soybean oil, cottonseed, safflower, sesame and sunflower oil. Excepting cashews and coconuts, most nuts are polyunsaturated. Polyunsaturated fats are so soft that they do not solidify even when chilled, as opposed to saturated fats. Because polyunsaturates lack the high cholesterol levels of saturated fats, many medical professionals believe they should be the main source of fat in the diet. Be advised, however, that opinions do vary on this issue. 'Polyunsaturated fats are not excreted by the body as efficiently as other fats,' asserts clinical nutritionist Dr Jairo Rodriguez. 'It's the *mono-unsaturated* fats, like olive oil and peanut oil, that

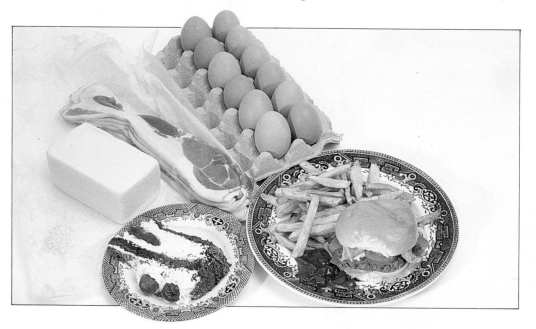

Eggs, meat, potatoes, cream and butter *(left)* all contain a high level of saturated fat. All saturated fat contains cholesterol. The presence of too much cholesterol in the bloodstream can lead to a dangerous heart condition and possibly a heart attack.

are the easiest for the body to break down and digest.' If you're still unsure about how much and what kind of fats you should be eating, remember that you can lower your chances of developing high cholesterol and heart disease by simply lowering your overall fat intake and obtaining more of your energy from other food sources, such as fruits and vegetables.

Why Your Body Needs Fibre

Fibre is the indigestible parts of food that stimulate the muscles of the large intestines, making bowel action more regular and easier. The necessity of fibre to our daily diet has been confirmed by recent medical studies, and many have concluded that lack of it contributes to constipation, haemorrhoids, diverticular disease (when the bowel becomes obstructed), cancer of the colon, heart disease and even varicose veins. Because we live in an age of chemically process-

ed, refined foods that are low in fibre, many of us have sluggish digestive systems. You can strengthen yours by making sure to eat a full ounce of fibre a day. Excellent sources include unprocessed bran flakes, stone ground grains (in breads or crackers), raw fruits and vegetables (with skins), and fresh squeezed, unstrained citrus juices. Additionally, if you substitute brown rice for white, you'll be getting much more fibre as a result.

Water: The Source

Water accounts for about 72 to 75 per cent of your total body weight. Dr Rodriguez counsels everyone to try to drink six to eight glasses of water a day, in addition to other fluid intake. 'There is no substitute for the compound that is water', he explains. 'Your body needs water more than it needs other liquids, and contrary to popular belief you will never become bloated from drinking too much water. By drinking lots of water, you will simply increase the efficiency of your body's water excretion, which can only do you good.' Maintaining a sufficient water balance is especially important for women, Dr Rodriguez adds, because water intake can help diminish pre-menstrual bloating. Of course, uncarbonated mineral water is healthier for you than tap water, which often contains impurities, so try to drink it whenever possible.

Brown rice, raw fruit, vegetables and breads *(below)* are all excellent sources of fibre. A diet high in fibre will improve the efficiency of your digestive system.

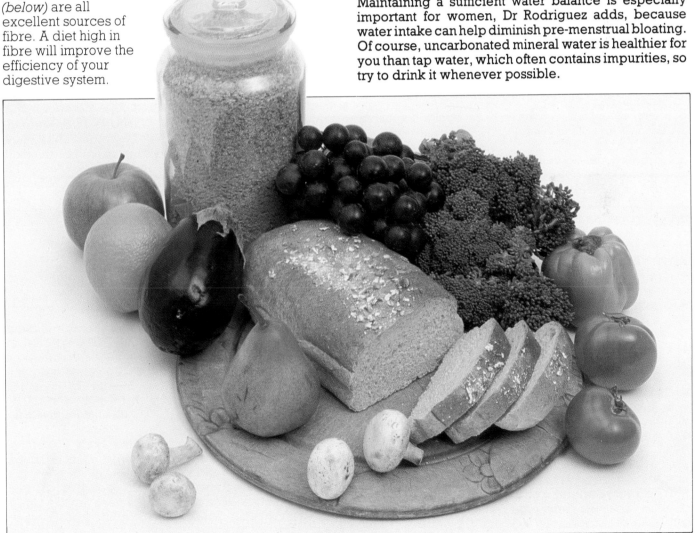

Vitamins and Minerals: What You Need to Know

Relatively complex, organic substances that occur naturally in plant and animal tissue, vitamins are essential in small amounts for the maintenance of the body's metabolic process. Deficiency of any one vitamin can lead to disease; conversely, '...overdosing on vitamin supplements can cause all manner of damage to the body', according to Dr Jairo Rodriguez. He strongly warns against following generalized vitamin supplement guidelines found in diet books, health food store literature and the like. Experimenting with your body in this way can waste your money, or even worse, endanger your health. To determine which vitamin and mineral supplements you may need, consult with a clinical nutritionist, discuss your medical history with them and have a blood analysis taken. If any deficiencies are found to exist, your doctor will be able to prescribe supplements accordingly.

Minerals are inorganic substances, such as iron, calcium and phosphorus. Several of them are essential to our diet, especially in the infant and childhood years. Certain non-dietary factors can influence the body's absorption and retention of vitamins and minerals. Here is just a sample:

- Every cigarette you smoke depletes your body of 25 milligrams of vitamin C.
- If you often take laxatives, you could be losing excessive amounts of potassium.
- Oral contraceptives, depending on the prescription, may sometimes increase the level of cholesterol in your blood. Some women have also been known to develop vitamin B-6 deficiency, which causes depression, as a result of taking birth control pills over a period of time.
- If you eat a lot of carbohydrates every day and drink alcohol often as well, you will most likely need extra vitamin B-1 to help metabolize food energy.
- Even if you are a light drinker, you may be deficient in the B vitamins and folic acid.
- Eating a diet high in refined carbohydrates, or processed foods in general, often leads to a deficiency in vitamin B-1.
- People who take aspirin regularly often suffer from iron deficiency. The reason is because aspirin irritates the lining of the stomach, triggering small but repeated loss of blood in the bowels.
- Some vitamins, such as those in the B-complex and vitamin C, lose much of their value when cooked or exposed to sunlight. Because many of the vitamins in fruits and vegetables are water soluble and heat sensitive, it's a good idea to re-program your preparation methods so that you get the full nutritional benefit from your food. You can do this by either lightly steaming your produce for a few minutes, or by eating fruits and vegetables raw in salads.

The Functions and Sources of Vitamins and Minerals

Vitamin A (also known as Retinol). Essential for good vision in dim light. A deficiency can cause night blindness. Helps protect the body's mucous membranes and reduces susceptibility to infection. Helps promote the growth and healing of glands, bones, teeth, nails and hair. Necessary for healthy, clear skin. Fat-soluble. *Natural sources:* Fish liver oils, butter, margarine, liver, kidneys, carrots and green vegetables like spinach and watercress.

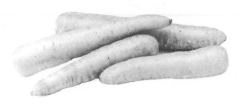

Vitamin B includes a complex of 11 vitamins; all of them play vital roles in the conversion of food into energy. Essential for the normal functioning of the nervous system and the maintenance of good digestion, the B-complex vitamins also help develop healthy skin, hair and eyes. These are water-soluble vitamins, which means they cannot be stored by your body and must be replaced every day. *Natural Sources:* Eggs, Brewer's yeast, liver and whole grain cereals.

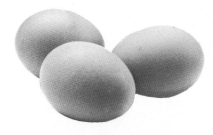

Vitamin B-1 (Thiamin). Essential for efficient digestion. Required for protein and carbohydrates to be used for energy. Also necessary for maintaining a healthy nervous system. Alcohol can cause deficiencies of this and all the other B-complex vitamins. *Natural Sources:* Wheat germ, Brewer's yeast, liver, whole grain cereals.

Vitamin B-2 (Riboflavin). Helps body to obtain energy from major nutrients. Helps maintain good vision and healthy skin. B-2 is resistant to heat, but sunlight destroys it (particularly in the case of milk and cheese). *Natural Sources:* Milk, cheese, lentils, eggs, all organ meats. Also, whole grain breads, and vegetables.

Vitamin B-4 (Niacin). Promotes utilization of protein, fats and carbohydrates. Necessary for a healthy nervous system and skin. Deficiency can cause pellagra, a disease where the skin becomes dark, tough and scaly. *Natural Sources:* Lean meats, poultry, fish, peanuts, Brewer's yeast, mushrooms and other vegetables. B-4 is unaffected by canning, cooking or freezing.

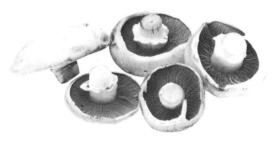

Vitamin B-6 (Pyridoxine). Essential for the production of red blood cells, nerve tissues, antibodies and the utilization of protein. Oral contraceptives can lower the body's levels of B-6; women who take them must supplement their diets with B-6 vitamins. Drinking alcohol also depletes your body of this vitamin. *Natural Sources:* Meats, liver, whole grains, green leafy vegetables and bananas.

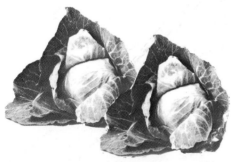

Vitamin B-12 Necessary for the normal development of red blood cells, and for the functioning of all cells, especially in the nervous system, bone marrow and intestines. Animal protein is the sole source of this vitamin, so vegetarians must obtain B-12 through either vitamin supplements or dairy products. B-12 can be stored in the liver. *Natural Sources:* All meat and dairy products.

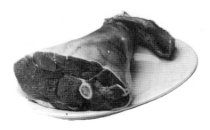

Folic Acid Essential for producing red blood cells and for maintaining normal metabolism. A deficiency can cause a form of anaemia. Drinking alcohol and taking oral contraceptives can deplete your body of folic acid. *Natural Sources:* Green leafy vegetables, liver, Brewer's yeast.

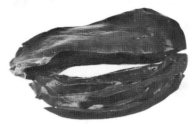

Biotin Vital to the digestive system, biotin also promotes healthy skin and hair. *Natural Sources:* Milk, egg yolk, Brewer's Yeast, beef liver and whole grains.

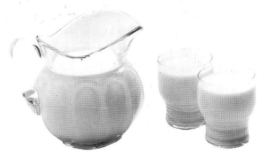

Pantothenic Acid Helps release energy from the major nutrients and supports a variety of body functions, including the maintenance of the nervous and digestive systems. *Natural Sources:* Can be found in almost all types of food, but can be destroyed by cooking and canning. Liver, kidney, vegetables, egg yolk, whole grains and Brewer's yeast.

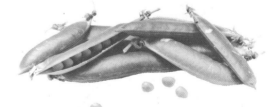

Para-aminobenzoic Acid (PABA). Necessary for healthy skin and hair pigmentation. Helps convert protein into energy. Promotes formation of red blood cells. *Natural Sources:* Molasses, wheat germ and liver.

Choline An element found in lecithin, which helps emulsify dietary fat. Also, choline aids in the transmission of nerve impulses. *Natural Sources:* Lecithin, egg yolks, liver, wheat germ and Brewer's yeast.

Inositol An important element in B-complex vitamins which helps convert food to energy. With choline, inositol is active in the metabolism of fats. *Natural Sources:* Unprocessed whole grain, Brewer's yeast and crude molasses.

Vitamin C (Ascorbic Acid). Promotes body's absorption of iron. Strengthens capillaries and other blood vessels. Controls the production of collagen, the connective material of all body tissues. Promotes healing of injuries and resistance to infection. Necessary for the health of teeth and gums. Vitamin C is water-soluble; it cannot be stored by the body and must be frequently replaced. *Natural sources:* Citrus fruits and juices, green peppers, strawberries and tomatoes.

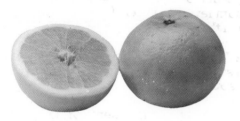

Vitamin D (Calciferol). Necessary for the body to absorb calcium and phosphorus. Essential for infants and growing children to ensure that teeth and bones develop properly. *Natural Sources:* Eggs, margarine, butter, fatty fish, liver. Sunlight acts upon the skin to form the vitamin in the body; D can be stored in the body.

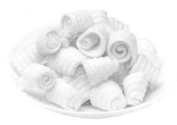

Vitamin E (Tocopherol). Necessary for the proper use of oxygen by the muscles. Acts as a preservative and tissue protector. Prolongs the life of red blood cells. *Natural Sources:* Fish, eggs, vegetable oils, wheat germ, whole grains, green vegetables, seeds and nuts.

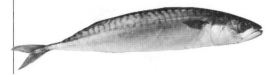

Calcium The most common mineral in the body. Essential for the formation and repair of bones and teeth. Also promotes the efficiency of nerves, muscle tone and blood clotting. *Natural Sources:* Milk and milk products, green leafy vegetables, citrus fruits, dried peas and beans, fish such as sardines where the bones are eaten.

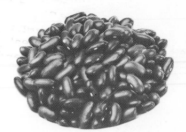

Chromium Aids in the metabolism of sugars into glucose, the form in which the body utilizes carbohydrates. Chromium is a trace element. *Natural Sources:* Seafood, unprocessed bran, whole grain cereals, Brewer's yeast and liver.

Cobalt Forms part of the B-12 molecule. A trace element. Strengthens control of metabolism, red blood cells and spinal cord. *Natural Sources:* Whole grain cereals, green vegetables, fruit and meat.

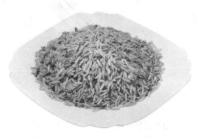

Copper Active in the storage and release of iron to form haemoglobin for red blood cells. *Natural Sources:* Organ meats, shellfish, nuts and dried legumes.

Fluoride A trace element which is often added to the water supply. Essential for strong tooth enamel, helps fight tooth decay. *Natural Sources:* Seafood. You can supplement your fluoride intake by taking fluoride tablets and brushing with fluoride toothpastes.

Iodine Necessary for the thyroid gland hormone and proper growth. Deficiency causes goitre, or swelling of the thyroid gland. Iodine is a trace element. *Natural sources:* Iodized salt (sea salt), seafood, kelp, tap water supply.

Iron A vital part of haemoglobin, a protein structure which aids red blood cells in transporting oxygen throughout the body. Deficiency causes the most common form of anaemia. Teenagers need extra iron during their years of maximum growth. Women need extra iron during the years when they are menstruating and especially during pregnancy. Recommended daily intake varies from 12 to 18 milligrams per day; the average diet contains approximately 12 milligrams. *Natural Sources:* Lamb's liver is the best source — 12.6 mg per 3oz (85 grams). Also, chicken liver, meat, eggs, green vegetables, dried apricots, cereal products, curry powder and cocoa. Iron from liver and meats is absorbed more efficiently than from any other sources.

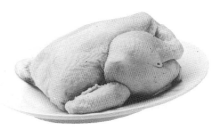

Magnesium Helps body absorb and use calcium and phosphorus. Promotes bone growth and is necessary for proper functioning of nerves and muscles. *Natural Sources:* Lentils, green vegetables, beans, seeds and nuts.

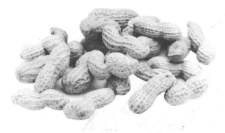

Manganese Promotes the development of normal tendon and bone structure. *Natural sources:* Bran, coffee, tea, kidneys, lentils, almonds, apricots, wheat germ and watercress.

Phosphorus Strengthens bones and teeth. Helps body obtain energy from food; phosphorus is found in every cell in our bodies. *Natural Sources:* Eggs, cheese, yeast, meat, chicken, fish and liver.

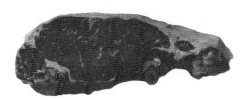

Potassium Vital to the normal functioning of the nervous system and muscles. The body excretes potassium frequently; there's a constant need for replenishment. Helps regulate body's water balance. *Natural Sources:* Dried apricots, baked potatoes, lima beans, bananas, milk, cheese, seafood and spinach.

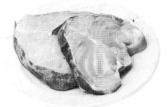

Selenium Interactive in the body with vitamin E. Low soil-selenium levels in parts of the world can result in depletion of this element.

Sodium Maintains balance of fluids in the body. Excessive salt intake may lead to high blood pressure in some people. Salt is in seafood, flavourings, dairy products, meat, fish, and especially processed foods. The minimum daily requirement for sodium can be satisfied by eating just a medium sized carrot and a stalk of celery! Most nutritionists advise the public to monitor their salt intake, as it can be a very unhealthful substance in high quantities.

Sulphur Aids in the formation of body tissues. *Natural Sources:* Nuts, beans, meat, cheese, eggs and fish.

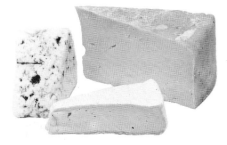

Zinc Important for respiration, growth, sexual development, tissue repair. Animal proteins are the best zinc sources, so vegetarians must remember to include zinc or zinc supplements in their diets. *Natural Sources:* Meat, fish, egg yolks, milk, whole grain cereals.

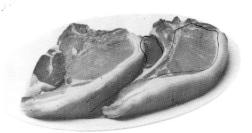

How to Fulfil Your Daily Nutritional Requirements

Now that you're familiar with the body's essential vitamin and mineral requirements and the specific foods that satisfy them, it's a good idea to pinpoint your eating habits to see what you can eat more (or less) of for improved nutrition. The checklist below will give you additional information on the quality of your diet.

1 Do you eat white bread and other refined flour products? You should know that white bread and other refined flours have had the wheat germ and bran removed, and are therefore much less nutritious than whole grained breads. White enriched bread has only three of the 11 vitamin B-complex added, whereas whole grained breads contain the whole B-complex and many other nutrients. Substitute all white flour products with whole grained ones and you'll not only feel more satisfied at mealtimes, but your body will become more enriched as well.

2 How much sugar do you eat in a day? Many nutritionists, Dr Rodriguez among them, suggest that you restrict your sugar intake to *natural sources only*. This means fresh fruits, vegetables and starches. Learn to live without white sugar, honey, maple syrup and brown sugar. Your body will thank you for it by operating more smoothly.

3 'Alcohol, because of its high sugar content and the fact that it is a central nervous system depressant, is a major insult to the body', says Dr Rodriguez. Besides being empty calories, it also depletes the vitamins and minerals stored in your body. If you are a regular drinker, reconsider your habit.

4 By now, you know what saturated fats can do to your body. If you want to safeguard your health, then reduce your overall fat intake. Also remember that fried foods are also considered by nutritionists to be a major insult to the body; you should avoid them from now on — they're a strain on the digestive system besides being fattening.

Colourful vegetables, such as carrots, are an important source of vitamin A. Carrots also contain vitamin E.

Green leafy vegetables such as cabbage provide vitamins A, B, C, E and K as well as iron, iodine and other valuable minerals.

Most fruits, particularly citrus fruits, are rich in vitamin C and the sugars in fruits are an instant and natural source of energy.

Wholemeal grains provide essential roughage for the digestive system and are a valuable source of vitamins B, E and K, as well as minerals.

5 The American National Research Council has established the Recommended Daily Allowance (RDA) for basic nutrients. Although the Council suggests that you eat two meat food groups a day, there is no reason why vegetarians cannot obtain their protein from other sources and have even better nutrition and health than meat eaters. After all, recent studies have shown that vegetarians often have denser bones than meat eaters! Besides needing two protein sources a day, however, you also require two or more cups of milk and milk products, and four or more servings of vegetables and fruits. Dark green or deep yellow vegetables should be eaten every other day; leafy green vegetables should be eaten as often as you like. The Council also advises that you eat citrus fruits every day. The last food group you need nutrients from is breads and cereals. Make yours whole grained for maximum fibre and nutritional value; eat four or more servings a day.

6 Don't forget that you need six to eight glasses of water each day, and in hot and humid weather you'll require more. A healthy diet requires constant replenishment of water, particularly if you take rigorous exercise.

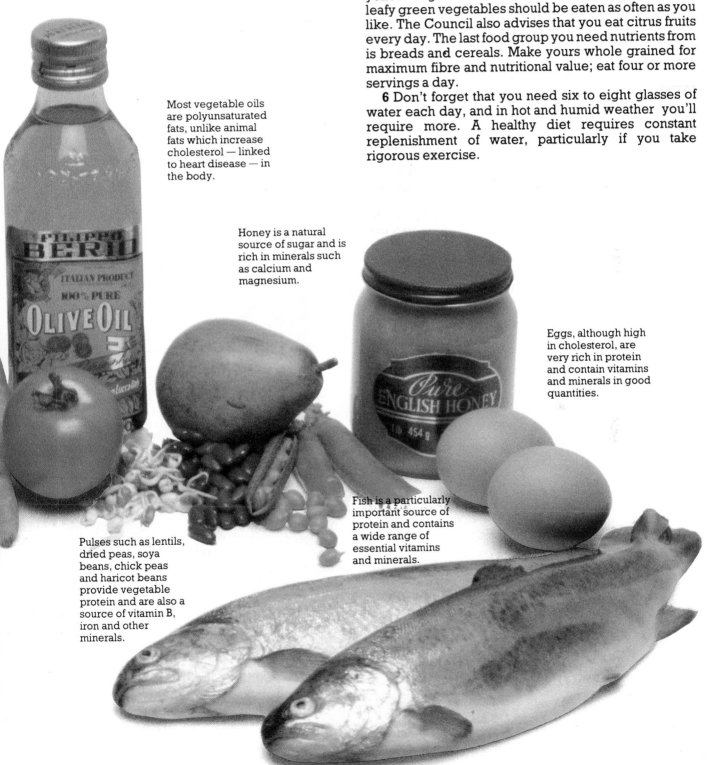

Most vegetable oils are polyunsaturated fats, unlike animal fats which increase cholesterol — linked to heart disease — in the body.

Honey is a natural source of sugar and is rich in minerals such as calcium and magnesium.

Eggs, although high in cholesterol, are very rich in protein and contain vitamins and minerals in good quantities.

Fish is a particularly important source of protein and contains a wide range of essential vitamins and minerals.

Pulses such as lentils, dried peas, soya beans, chick peas and haricot beans provide vegetable protein and are also a source of vitamin B, iron and other minerals.

7 Do you eat processed foods containing preservatives, artificial colouring and/or flavouring? If you do, eliminate them completely from your diet! No food that has been chemically altered is good for you.

8 Do you eat *only* when you're hungry? Do you plan all of your meals carefully so that you obtain the nutrients you need? If you're not in the habit of doing so, now is the time to begin. Better nutrition will improve your energy level and prepare your body for the exercise programs detailed in the following chapters.

Diet Plans and Snacks for Building Energy and Muscle

Let's assume you are preparing to start this book's exercise program but are slightly overweight, or, that you simply need to re-educate your eating habits. If you follow the 1,000 calorie a day menus listed below, they'll help you lose what you want and make exercising easier for you. These meal plans give both the calories of separate dishes as well as the total intake for the meal, so you can see what your daily calorie count will be and make substitutions if you like. You may want to buy a paperback calorie and carbohydrate counter so that you can plan more personalized meals; if you want to be a purist, you can also pick up a pocket book *sodium* counter to monitor your salt intake.

Breakfasts

1. 5 fluid oz (140ml) orange juice — 45 calories
    1 egg, boiled or poached — 80 calories
    1 slice whole wheat bread, lightly buttered — 100 calories
    coffee with milk — 20 calories

    TOTAL: 245 calories

Lunches

1. ¼lb (113 grams) sliced white turkey — 199 calories
    small mixed salad — 20 calories
    lemon and vinegar dressing — 13 calories
    ½ cup strawberries (75mg) — 28 calories

    TOTAL: 260 calories

2. ½ medium avocado (pitted) — 167 calories
    stuffed with 1 small diced tomato, onion and parsley — 50 calories
    ½ cup blueberries — 45 calories

    TOTAL: 262 calories

3. ¼lb (113 grams) calf's liver (broiled) garnished with tomato; onion slices — 158 calories
    black coffee — none

    TOTAL: 173 calories

Dinners

1. 8oz (226 grams) broiled chicken on the bone — do not eat skin! — 200 calories
    6 asparagus spears — 60 calories
    3oz (85 grams) black grapes — 45 calories

    TOTAL: 305 calories

2. ¼lb (113 grams) broiled haddock; garnished with lime juice and chives — 179 calories
    lettuce, cucumber, mushroom salad with garlic, vinegar and lemon — 70 calories
    1 pear — 40 calories

    TOTAL: 289 calories

3. 5oz (140 grams) steamed whitefish, garnished with lemon juice and mushrooms — 135 calories
    1 small baked potato — 120 calories
    1 cup unsweetened apple juice — 117 calories

    TOTAL: 372 calories

4. 4oz (115 grams) halibut, broiled in lemon — 170 calories
    spinach, mushroom and yellow squash salad — 60 calories
    lemon, garlic and vinegar dressing
    6oz (170 grams) slice melon — 25 calories

    TOTAL: 255 calories

Keep in mind, if and when you are dieting, that restricting your intake to certain food groups will have a 'fine tuning' effect on the digestive system. Your stomach could be seriously upset if you suddenly resume eating many foods that you have abstained from for some time. Anything fried or fatty, sugary desserts, meat dishes and alcohol are some obvious examples of hard-to-digest substances. So, when coming off a diet, it's a good idea to gradually reintroduce yourself to the foods you've foregone in order to lose weight.

This nutritional chart of the protein, calorie, carbohydrate and fat content of common, healthful foods comes courtesy of Lydia Cheng, a top professional bodybuilder who trains in New York and Paris.

FOOD	MEASURE	PROTEIN	CALORIES	CARBS	FAT
BREADS:					
cracked wheat	1 slice	2grams	60	12	.6
French	1 slice	1.8	50	11.1	.64
pumpernickel	1 slice	2.9	79	17	.4
rye	1 slice	2.1	56	12	.3
white	1 slice	2.0	62	11.6	.79
whole wheat	1 slice	2.4	56	11.0	.7
cream of wheat	1 cup	4.5	133	28.2	.4
granola (Nature's V)	1 cup	9.0	390	57.0	15.0
oatmeal	1 cup	4.8	132	23.3	2.4
macaroni, cooked	1 cup	4.8	151	32.2	1.0
popcorn	1 cup	1.6	54	10.7	.7
bran muffin	1 avg (40g)	3.1	104	17.2	3.9
corn muffin	1 avg (45g)	3.2	130	19.1	4.6
rice — brown, dry	1 cup	14.8	704	152	3.6
rice — white, dry	1 cup	13.1	708	157	1.5
wheat germ	1 cup	26.6	363	46.7	10.9
EGGS:					
raw, extra large	1	7.4	94	.5	7.24
raw, large	1	6.5	82	.5	6.44
raw, medium	1	5.7	72	.4	5.65
raw, small	1	5.2	65	.4	4.5
raw, white	1 large	3.6	17	.3	0
raw, yolk	1 large	2.79	59	.1	5.7
FISH:					
cod	1 lb	79.8	354	0	3.31
crab	"	78.5	422	2.3	8.6
flounder, sole	"	75.8	358	0	8.6
haddock	"	83.0	358	0	2.90
halibut	"	94.8	454	0	4.98
lobster	"	76.7	413	2.3	8.6
scallops	"	69.4	367	15.0	.9
shrimp	"	82.1	413	6.8	3.6
snapper	"	89.8	422	0	5.44
tuna (water)	"	56.0	254	0	1.6
FRUIT/FRUIT JUICES:					
apple	1 med. (150g)	.3	96	24.0	1
dried apple	1 cup	.9	234	61.0	1.4
apple juice	1 cup	.2	117	29.5	t
applesauce	1 cup	.5	100	26.4	.5
avocado, pitted	1 avg	4.2	334	12.6	32.8
banana, raw	1 avg	1.6	127	33.3	.3

FOOD	MEASURE	PROTEIN	CALORIES	CARBS	FAT
blackberries	1 cup	1.7	84	18.6	1.3
blueberries	1 cup	1.0	90	22.2	.7
canteloupe	¼ avg	.7	30	7.5	.1
cherries. pitted	1 cup	1.9	90	22.2	.5
grapefruit, raw	½ med	.5	41	10.8	.1
grapefruit juice, raw	1 cup	1.2	98	23.0	.2
grapes	1 cup	2.0	106	24.0	1.5
honeydew melon	150mg	1.2	49	11.5	t
nectarine, raw	1 avg	.8	88	23.6	t
orange	1 avg	1.3	64	16.0	.3
orange juice, unsw.	1 cup	1.7	112	25.8	.5
papaya, raw	½ med	.9	58	15	.15
peach, raw	1 med	.6	38	9.7	.1
pear	1 avg	1.4	122	30.6	.8
pear, dried	1 cup	5.6	482	121.0	3.2
pineapple, raw	1 cup	.6	81	21.2	.3
plums, raw	2 med	.5	66	17.8	t
prunes, dried	1 cup (185mg)	3.4	411	108.0	1
raisins, packed	1 cup	4.1	477	128.0	.3
raspberries, black	1 cup	2.0	98	21.0	1.9
raspberries, red	1 cup	1.5	70	16.7	.6
raspb. juice, unsw.	1 cup	t	49	12.8	0
strawberries	1 cup (150mg)	1	56	12.6	.8
tangelo, raw	1 med	.5	39	9.2	.1
tangerine	1 med	.7	39	10.0	.2
watermelon, cubes	1 cup	.5	26	6.4	.2
MEAT & POULTRY:					
beef:					
ground beef, lean	1 lb	93.9	812	0	45.4
liver	1 lb	90.3	635	24.0	17.3
round steak	1 lb	88.5	863	0	53.9
sirloin steak	1 lb	71	1316	0	112
chicken:					
breast	1 lb	74.5	394	0	112
duck	1 lb	59.5	1213	0	130
turkey — light	1 lb	149	798	0	17.7
turkey — dark	1 lb	136	921	0	37.6
VEGETABLES:					
alfalfa sprouts	100g	5.1	41	0	.6
asparagus — pieces	1 cup	3.4	35	6.8	.3
asparagus — spears	4	2.2	20	3.6	.2
green beans, raw	1 cup	2.1	35	7.8	1.2
soybean sprouts, raw	1 cup	6.5	48	5.6	1.5
broccoli, cooked	1 cup	4.8	40	7	.5
brussels sprouts	9 med	4.9	45	8.3	.4

cabbage, common, raw	1 cup	.9 (70g)	17	3.8	.1
cabbage, chinese, raw	1 cup	.9	11	2.3	.1
carrots	1 large	9.7	42	9.7	.2
cauliflower, raw	1 cup	2.7	27	5.2	.2
celery, raw	1 cup	1.1	20	4.7	.1
corn, cooked	1 cup	5.3	137	31	1.7
cucumber. raw, sliced	1 cup	.9	16	3.6	.1
eggplant, cooked	1 cup (200g)	2	38	8.2	.4
endive, raw	1 cup (50g)	.9	10	2.1	.1
ginger root	3.5oz	1.4	49	9.5	1.0
leeks, raw	3-4	2.2	52	11.2	.3
lettuce, boston or bib	1 cup	.7	8	1.4	.1
lettuce, iceberg	1 cup	.7	10	2.2	.1
mushrooms, raw	1 cup (70g)	1.9	20	3.1	.2
onions, raw	1 cup (170g)	2.6	65	14.8	.2
parsley, raw	1 cup (60g)	2.2	26	5.1	.4
peas, raw	1 cup (145g)	9.1	122	20.9	.6
peppers, green, raw	1 cup (80g)	1	18	3.8	.2
potato, raw, diced	1 cup (150g)	3.2	114	25.7	.2
potato, baked (skin)	1 large (202g)	4	145	32.5	.2
potato, boiled (skin)	1 med (100g)	2.1	76	17.1	.1
radish	10 med (50g)	.5	8	1.6	t
spinach, raw	1 cup (55g)	1.8	14	2.4	.2
squash, summer, raw	1 cup (130g)	1.4	25	5.5	.1
winter squash	1 cup (205g)	3.7	129	31.6	.8
sweet potato, baked	1 avg (146g)	2.4	161	37	.6
tomato, raw	1 med (150g)	1.6	33	7	.3
tomatoes, canned	1 cup	2.4	51	10.4	.5
tomatoes, juice	1 cup	2.2	46	10.4	.2
watercress, raw	1 cup (35g)	.8	7	1.1	.1

Weights and Measures:
1 microgram = 1/1,000,000 gram
1,000 micrograms = 1 milligram
1 milligram = 1/1,000 gram
1,000 milligrams = 1 gram
1.00 oz = 28.35 grams
3.57 oz = 100 grams
0.25 lb = 113.00 grams
0.50 lb = 227.00 grams
1.00 lb = 453.00 grams

1 quart = 4 cups
1 pint = 2 cups
1 cup = ½ pint
1 cup = 8 fluid oz, or 16 tablespoons
2 tblsp. = 1 fluid oz
1 tblsp. = 3 tsp.

1 avg serving = 4 oz
1 oz fluid = 28 grams

1 cup fluid:
    cooking oil = 200 grams
    water = 220 grams
    milk, soups = 240 grams

1 cup, dry:
    cereal flakes = 50 grams
    flours = 100 grams
    sugars = 200 grams

High Sodium
tomatoes
celery
carrots
broccoli
spinach

Lean Fish
haddock, halibut and cod

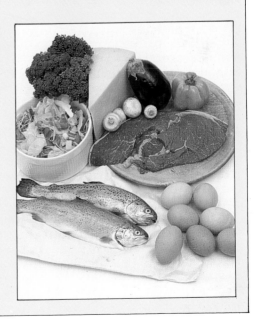

Chapter 2
Getting your body in gear

All About Muscles

As has been previously mentioned, there are inherent differences between men's and women's bodies. Because men carry about 25 per cent fewer fat cells than women, they are innately more muscular. A man's naturally larger bone structure not only gives him extra strength, but the male hormone testosterone allows for much greater muscular growth than the average woman can hope to achieve. Physical limitations aside, however, women excel in endurance, and are capable of developing overall muscular strength that is comparably equal to a man's. Women's extra layer of fatty tissue between the muscles and the skin makes them superior to men in sports like long distance swimming; research by exercise physiologists has found that women are just as physically qualified as men to undertake a weight training/bodybuilding program.

There are three types of major muscle tissue in the body. Each type differs in structure, location, function and activation. Smooth muscle lies in the walls of internal or visceral organs such as the intestines and blood vessels. We cannot control these muscles, as they work automatically. Weight training can benefit these muscles because it stimulates blood circulation and oxygen flow throughout the body. Examples of smooth muscle include the uterus, oesophagus and intestinal muscles.

Cardiac, or heart muscles become stronger through exercise which increases the heart rate. Although weight training can strengthen your heart, swimming, running and cycling will give you more cardiovascular improvement in less time.

Skeletal muscle is the assortment of long muscles that control physical coordination and movement. This type of muscle grows stronger and larger through various kinds of programmed exercise, but you'll achieve increased muscularity quickest by progressive resistance (weight training) exercise that involves more and more poundage over time. Although it's a fact that general skeletal and muscle structure is the same for everyone, all bodies are different and some have better genetic potential for developing strength than others. The good news is that no matter what Nature gave you, you can build on it as much as you like, strengthening and re-shaping your body through conscientious diet and careful exercise.

General Facts about Weight Training and Bodybuilding

Many people confuse weight training and body-building with *weight lifting*. These are two decidedly different sports. Weightlifters train with extremely heavy weights to become as strong as possible, while keeping their weight within the limits of their particular competitive class. Weight training and bodybuilding have aesthetic as well as athletic goals; these results are achieved through the synchronized use of weights to shape, strengthen and condition the body in an integrated way. Just because you start training with weights does not mean you will attain a competitive bodybuilder's unusually well developed physique. Many bodybuilders who have been training seriously for years never work with heavy weights, as they prefer to stay lean and trim. Since a competitive bodybuilder trains up to five hours a day for years on end and follows a controlled diet in order to achieve maximum muscularity, there is very little chance of a man or a woman becoming 'muscle bound' through a standard weight training program.

Bodybuilding and weight training work the muscles through what is known as 'progressive resistance' exercises. One of the simplest examples of this term is a classic push-up, where you lie face down on the floor, hands beside your shoulders, palms down, fingers forward. Only your toes rest on the floor to support your lower body; your heels are in the air. Keeping your body straight, you push up with your hands and arms until your elbows are nearly straight. Then you lower yourself until your chest brushes the floor. You exhale on the resistance part of the exercise (pushing up), and inhale on the relaxation phase (lowering yourself to the floor). The muscles undergoing resistance here are in the chest, shoulders and upper arms — each push-up

The skeletal muscles *(right)* control the physical coordination and movement of the body. The quickest way to achieve increased muscularity is through progressive resistance (weight training) exercise.

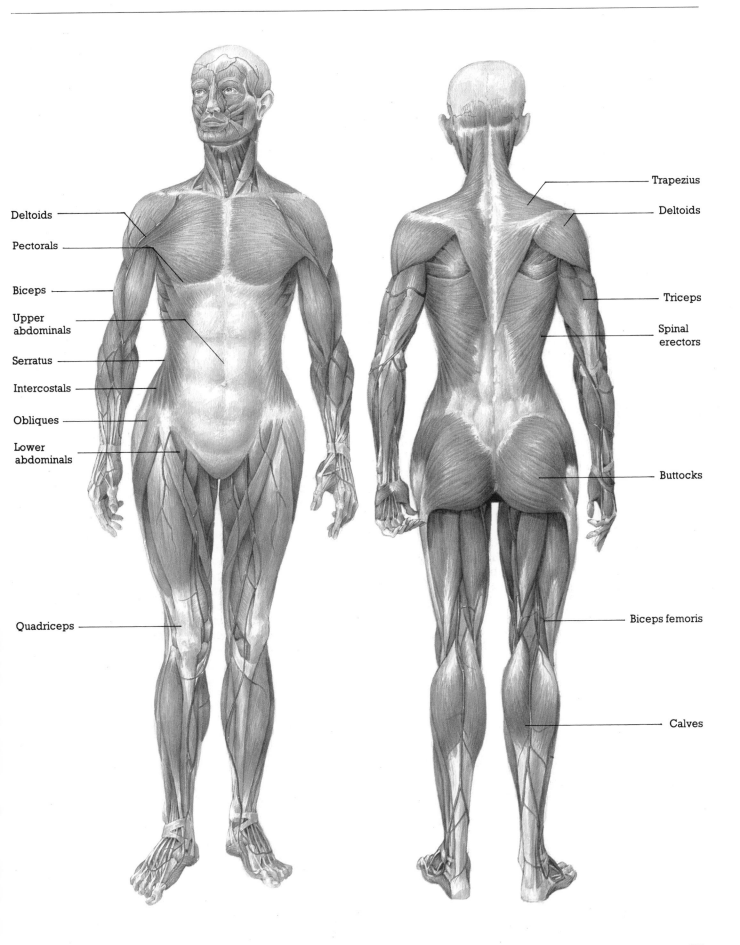

Deltoids

Pectorals

Biceps

Upper
abdominals

Serratus

Intercostals

Obliques

Lower
abdominals

Quadriceps

Trapezius

Deltoids

Triceps

Spinal
erectors

Buttocks

Biceps femoris

Calves

will increase the blood flow in these areas.

While progressive resistance exercises work isolated muscles in the body and increase the size and strength of muscle tissue, they will not decrease the amount of fat around the muscles. This is because weight training exercises are short term exercises that burn up *glucose* rather than fat calories. Weight training compels the body to use a lot of oxygen in a short period of time. At the end of a set of exercises you create an oxygen debt that must be repaid by resting from one to three minutes, depending on the intensity of the exercise. Whether you work your muscles strenuously through lifting weights or doing several push-ups or sit-ups, you'll know that you're getting the full benefit of the exercise when you feel the extra blood flowing in your muscles and swelling them up. This feeling is accompanied by a sense of well-being and is called a 'pump'. Because weight training and other forms of anaerobic exercise are extremely beneficial yet at the same time inefficient when it comes to burning off fat, you may want to know more about *aerobic* exercise and how it affects your metabolism.

Anaerobic and Aerobic Exercise

Exercise physiologists such as Dr Rodriguez recommend a combined program of anaerobic (weight training) and aerobic exercise (running, cycling, swimming) as being the quickest, most efficient route to weight loss and also to the development of lean muscle tissue.

The term aerobic means air, and refers to the oxygen in the air. Because muscles need oxygen to function, their oxygen need rises when you work them. Exercise physiologists define aerobic exercise as any endurance sport that demands steady, uninterrupted output from your muscles over 12 minutes or more. Why the 12 minute minimum? Research has proved that a 12 minute period of aerobic exercise is the minimum duration for producing the heart and muscle enzyme changes that can quicken your metabolism, causing you to burn more calories throughout the day, even while you sleep.

Now you know exactly how these two types of exercise affect the muscles and speed up the body's use of calories. If you exercise aerobically and do progressive resistance exercises three days a week, you can expect to lose weight while building leaner, stronger muscles. Of course, your diet will also affect the rate of your metabolism and accompanying weight loss. Exercising aerobically six days a week, coupled with weight training, will bring you even quicker, more dramatic results. Not only will you burn off pounds of fat, but your strength and fitness will be markedly improved.

It all depends on what your goals are, and how hard you want to work for them. No matter how out of shape you may be, today is the day you can begin re-shaping your body through careful diet and sensibly planned exercise.

Evaluating Your Fitness Level and Strength

To begin with, for safety's sake, you should obtain a doctor's permission for beginning the exercise plans in this book. Men over 40 and people with any heart problem must be especially careful; they should have a stress electrocardiogram test before starting any exercise program.

How do you judge if you're at a beginning, intermediate or advanced level? Thus far, only cardiovascular (aerobic) and progressive resistance (anaerobic) fitness have been explained here. There happens to be a third category of exercise that is a factor in one's overall fitness — stretching.

Stretching exercises are extremely helpful in warming up and relieving tension in a muscle before it is worked. Without flexible muscles and tendons, you risk injury even while doing the simplest of exercises. Accordingly, the following checklist has been devised to help you gauge your relative flexibility, strengths and weakness. Results will be based on your performance of particular exercises in all three categories of exercise.

Checklist for Women's Fitness

Progressive Resistance (Anaerobic) Fitness

Earlier, the push-up was cited as a classic illustration of progressive resistance movement. It also happens to be an excellent measure of the upper body's strength and muscular power. How many can you do? If you finish 15 or more repetitions, then you have superior upper body strength. If you can do five to 10 repetitions, you're about average. Anything less than five means that you need to work on building strength in your shoulders, triceps, pectorals and back.

To see how strong your legs are, try doing what is known as a wall sit. This mainly works the muscles in your thighs, the quadriceps. Position yourself against a wall, feet shoulder width apart, toes pointed straight ahead, feet roughly 18 to 24 inches from the wall, depending on your height. Lower yourself into a sitting position, as if you were seated on an invisible chair. Let your arms rest against the wall but *don't* use them to hold yourself up. Stay in this position for as long as you can. If you can go five minutes, consider yourself a champion! Most women, however, will probably find that they will only be able to hold this position for about a minute or two at first.

The push-up and wall sit exercises are both ideal for evaluating your fitness level and strength. The number of push-ups you can do and the length of time you can maintain the wall sit will determine the amount of work you need to do on your shoulders, triceps, pectorals, back and quadriceps *(right)*.

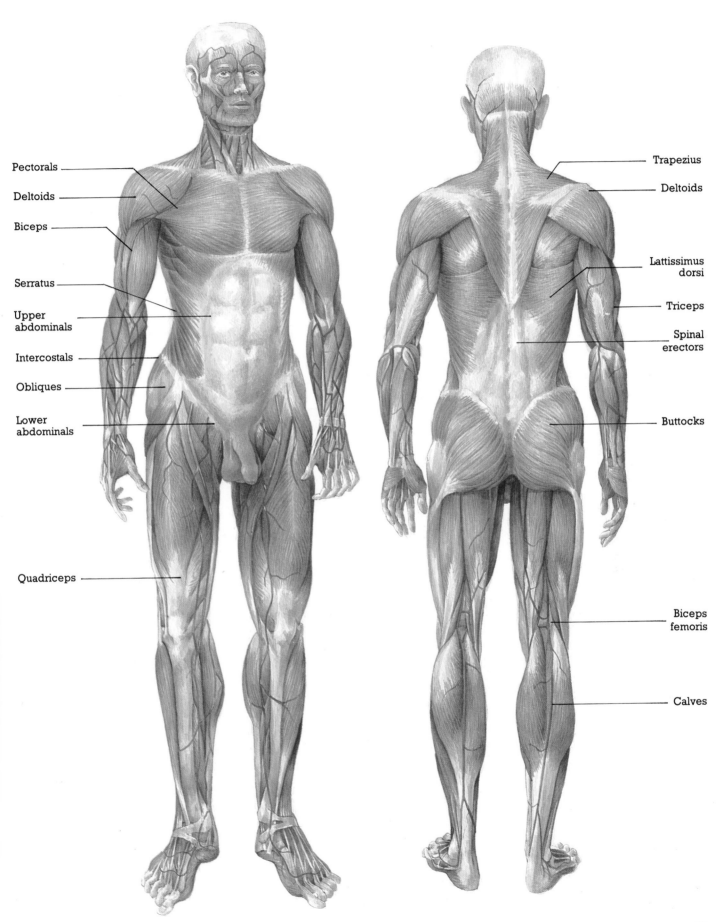

Pectorals

Deltoids

Biceps

Serratus

Upper
abdominals

Intercostals

Obliques

Lower
abdominals

Quadriceps

Trapezius

Deltoids

Lattissimus
dorsi

Triceps

Spinal
erectors

Buttocks

Biceps
femoris

Calves

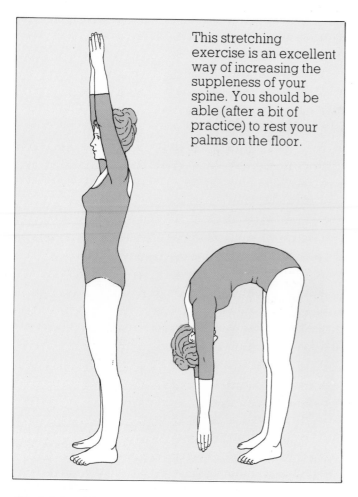

This stretching exercise is an excellent way of increasing the suppleness of your spine. You should be able (after a bit of practice) to rest your palms on the floor.

Stretching Fitness

With feet together, bend forward from the waist and touch your toes. If you can hold this position for a full minute without pain in your buttock, thigh or calf muscles, then you're all the more pre-conditioned for weight training and/or supplementary exercise programs.

Conversely, if your hands hover several inches above your feet and your muscles feel strained from the stretch, then you must practice improving your flexibility. Do the toe stretch every day with the goal of holding it for a minute or more. After mastering this, try stretching your palms all the way down to the floor, and hold them there for a minute. This is one of the best stretching exercises there is! Remember that the goal of stretching is maximum extension of the muscles and tendons for increased suppleness; never bounce while you stretch, as the motion will preclude elongation of the muscles and may cause injury. It's far wiser to stretch as far as you can for as long as you can, gradually increasing your flexibility.

To test back, shoulder and upper arm flexibility, lie on your stomach and chest with your head off the floor, arms lifted behind you and to the sides. Raise your legs and upper body as far as you can stretch, so that they move towards each other. Keep only your stomach and

hips on the floor. Hold this position for five seconds and slowly lower yourself to the floor. You should feel the stretch especially in the lower back and the back of the arms.

If you have to strain to hold this position, then you know how much you need to limber up before beginning weight training, or any other form of exercise. A supple lower back is positively *essential* for weight training, as the stress of progressive resistance exercise often involves the back muscles.

		Advised Heart Rates **Exercise During Aerobic**	
AGE	MAXIMUM HEART RATE	80% of Max. (Advised Training Rate)	75% of Max. (for those with heart disease history); NOT TO EXCEED:
20	200	160	150
22	198	158	148
24	196	157	147
26	194	155	145
28	192	154	144
30	190	152	143
32	189	151	142
34	187	159	140
36	186	149	140
38	184	147	138
40	182	146	137
45	179	143	134
50	175	140	131
55	171	137	128
60	160	128	120
65 and over	150	120	113

Cardiovascular (Aerobic) Fitness

Because aerobic workouts place such demands on the heart and lungs, it's crucial that you know how to exercise at a sensible level, without straining yourself. The effectiveness of aerobic exercise is gauged by measuring the oxygen demands of the muscles. As the oxygen demand increases, your heart rate moves faster and faster. As you exercise harder and harder, your heart rate moves faster and faster. As illustrated in the heart rate chart above, your heart rate reaches a maximum for your age which no amount of strenuous exercise can increase. To achieve substantial fitness gains, you should only exercise hard enough to make your heart go at 80 per cent of the maximum for your age.

Because it is impossible to define a standard level of aerobic fitness for people of different sexes, ages and health histories, it is far more useful to you to follow this method for evaluating the effectiveness of your aerobic exertions. Choose any of the aforementioned exercises that are steady, endurance aerobic sports. Exercise at the appropriate heart rate for at least 12 minutes, non-stop, six days a week. The first few sessions you should stop after a minute or two and take your pulse. Count your pulse beats with a watch for six seconds and multiply by 10 to get the beats per minute. If the pulse is less than your correct exercise rate, you aren't working out hard enough. If the pulse is too high, then slow down a bit. This simple method of measuring aerobic effectiveness is standard practice for coaches and athletes. It's called 'pulse-monitored training' and is the safest way to help get yourself in shape. The preceding chart is based on resting heart rates of 72 for males and 80 for females. Again, men over 40 and people with a heart problem are advised to have stress electrocardiogram tests before starting any exercise programs.

Following this program will ensure steady aerobic re-conditioning. Women should not for a moment be discouraged by initial weak performance in progressive resistance exercises, aerobic workouts, etc. Once you are in shape, you will find that your endurance grows and grows.

It is recommended that women start with the beginning program in this book, both for safety's sake and to familiarize themselves with the proper form and variations of weight training exercises. Whether your body requires intensive re-conditioning before and during your beginning weight training program, or if you simply want to increase strength, coordination and endurance, now you know *how* and *where* to begin. You may feel free to try some of the intermediate exercises, but *do be sensible* and don't strain your muscles beyond their abilities. Remember, it takes time to build strength!

Checklist for Men's Fitness

Progressive Resistance (Anaerobic Fitness)
If you can complete up to 15 push-ups in proper form, then you're probably most suited to begin with the intermediate exercise program in this book. If you can complete up to 5 repetitions, your conditioning would seem to be at the beginner's level. Doing 20 or more with proper form qualifies you as strong enough to begin with the advance section of exercises.

Also, try the wall sit exercise described in the women's checklist. You should be able to hold it for two minutes or more. If you cannot and it's a definite strain, then you obviously need to practice improving strength in your legs. You can do this by increasing the number of repetitions of leg exercises that are suggested, as well as by practicing the wall sit each day.

Stretching Fitness
See the women's checklist and try both exercises. If you cannot touch your toes, consider yourself in need of conditioning. Do stretching work each day, at least once. There's no reason why you can't take a minute from your work at the office and try stretching in the middle of the day. It'll rid you of tension and clear your head, besides getting your body in shape for weight training. As regards the upper body flexibility exercise, if you can do 20 of these then you're in fairly good condition and can probably start the intermediate exercises with ease. This movement is an excellent warm-up and strengthener. If you can only do a few, then do practice working up to 20 or more.

Cardiovascular (Aerobic) Fitness
Again, please read through the women's section for this. The only relevant difference between men and women regarding aerobic conditioning is that of resting heart rate — 72 for men and 80 for women. You can determine your advised rate of aerobic exertion by referring to the heart rate chart first.

After reviewing the above guidelines and fitness indicators, you should be able to make a fairly knowing appraisal of your physical condition. You're ready for the advanced exercises only if you're strong enough anaerobically and aerobically to work out at peak performance. If you're flexible as well, so much the better. Most of you are probably capable of starting with the intermediate section. If you have any obvious weaknesses or doubts, however, be careful and start at the beginning level. It doesn't take much time to work your way up to heavier weights once you find your groove.

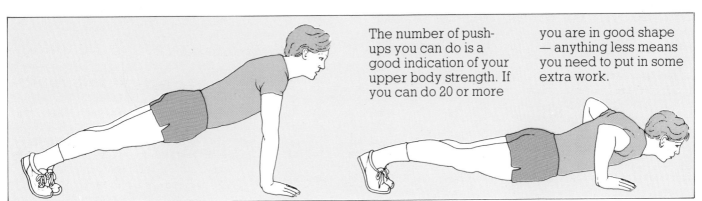

The number of push-ups you can do is a good indication of your upper body strength. If you can do 20 or more you are in good shape — anything less means you need to put in some extra work.

Underused Muscles:

How Building Certain Muscle Areas Can Improve Your Health

Some of the most commonly underused muscle areas are the back, stomach, buttocks, thighs and — especially with women — the upper arms. The average person's combination of unconditioned muscles often contributes to a host of minor ailments. For example, undeveloped muscles in the stomach and back can impair both your posture and breathing. Poor posture and inefficient breathing are two of the biggest causes of backaches, headaches and stiff necks. Weight training can eliminate problems like these by strengthening the vital muscle areas that affect your body's alignment and carriage.

John Perretti, the owner and manager of the New York gym Madison Avenue Muscle, puts it this way: 'A person who doesn't exercise much, whose back starts hurting and is generally out of shape — they probably need to develop muscle tone along the spine. Once they start training, their bodies will straighten themselves out — the body *wants* to be straight. After lifting weights for a short period, the spine moves into its true, correct lineage. So lifting and weight training can be a corrective for anyone who needs it.' John's associate, Patrick Arnao, also adds that he's seen cases where people suffering from chronic asthma lessened the severity of their symptoms through a steady program of weight training with free weights and machines.

These health benefits aside, however, there is also considerable evidence to prove that strengthening the upper and lower abdominal muscles through exercise increases the efficiency of your digestive organs. And it's a medically certified fact that the more strain that you relieve your inner organs of, the healthier your body will be.

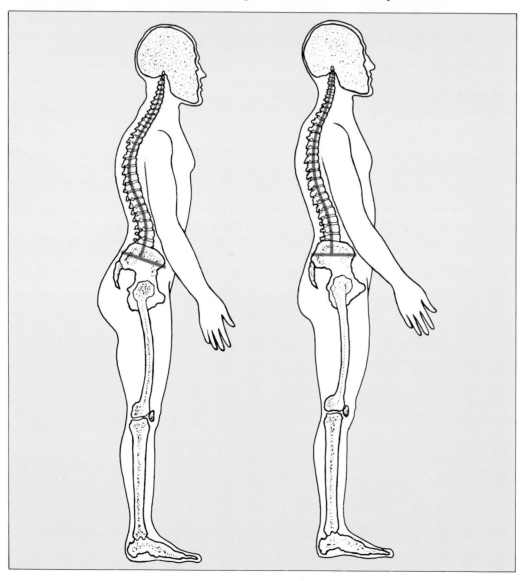

Undeveloped muscles in your stomach and back manifest themselves in poor posture and breathing *(far left)* By training with weights these vital muscle areas can be strengthened and will result in a much better posture *(left)*

How To Avoid And/Or Treat Injuries

First of all, when lifting free weights (dumb-bells or bar-bells) you must exercise proper form in breathing and controlling the weight so as to get maximum results from the movement. Proper breathing dictates that one inhales on the relaxation phase of the movement, and exhales on the resistance phase. Controlling the weight properly requires that both phases of the movement take the same amount of time, allowing the muscles to benefit from fully balanced stress and range of motion. That is to say, if it takes you five seconds to lower a dumb-bell as you do a biceps curl, then you should take five seconds raising it to your starting position. If you find that you have difficulty maintaining control of dumb-bells or barbells, you may want to try working out on exercise machines instead. These machines are designed to make it as easy as possible for the body to perform a specific movement. Machines have a built-in *groove*, so to speak, and they control your movement. With free weights, however, you have complete control, and your form can make the difference between a good workout and a great one. Maintaining proper form at all times is one of the surest ways to avoid muscle stress and injury.

It is equally important to make sure that your muscles are thoroughly warmed up before each workout. Always use the suggested body position described in each exercise! Experimenting with new positions of your own may lead to injury. Good training habits should also include careful attention to loose weights in your training area. Never leave them lying around on the floor, always return them to their respective racks or storage spaces.

To protect your back and other muscles from strain and injury, use a weightlifting belt when doing heavy back exercises, overhead lifts and squats. These belts are made from sturdy leather and can be bought in most sporting goods stores and gyms. Finally, if you are lifting heavy weights, or beginning to train seriously, you may want to consider finding a training partner to help you with your workouts. A partner can stand by and rescue you if, for instance, you fail to complete a heavy lift and are about to drop the barbell. A partner can keep an eye on your form and tell you when you may be cheating on a particularly strenuous movement. Additionally, if you are a beginner who is adjusting to the rigours of a new weight lifting program, a workout partner can help you overcome the initial mental and physical challenges that accompany this kind of exercise.

Before you work out, read through the descriptions of the exercises you'll be doing. Reread the descriptions while studying the accompanying photos of the exercises. Next, try using a broomstick to practice the exercise without weights. When you have run through the exercises and feel confident that you know what you're doing, you're ready to begin working out. Remember to start with light weights, increasing popularity only when there is a minimal exertion involved.

Many people lift weights without so much as a strained muscle. If you warm up thoroughly and then maintain a steady, rapid workout pace to keep your muscles warm; if you use proper positions and form in all exercises and lift sensibly chosen poundages, then you should remain injury-free. Nevertheless, should an accident happen, you must be prepared to handle routine training injuries. Beth Rubino, a competitive bodybuilder and model who trains six days a week, offers the following guidelines:

- If an injury is disabling, you should immediately go to a hospital emergency room, or to your personal physician, for attention. Severe strains and sprains, broken bones and dislocated joints need to be examined, X-rayed, etc as soon as possible.
- If you incur a muscle strain or a minor joint sprain (these are the most common bodybuilding injuries), your muscle will feel mildly sore or there will be pain in a specific area, such as the lower back. A minor injury like this is typically experienced as an increasing pain during a workout, followed by a steady — although mild — pain that you feel for several days afterwards.
- Even if you feel no pain in the muscle or joint a day after an injury, you should still be careful when doing movements involving the injured area. Reducing your normal poundage by 25 per cent will safeguard against further strain while giving the area a chance to regain its strength.
- More painful or serious injuries should be treated with ice (immediately) to prevent swelling. Rub the area with an ice cube for five minutes every hour or two, depending on how painful it is.

A day and a half to two days after the injury, you should apply a hot water bottle wrapped in a damp towel to the area. Damp heat is more easily absorbed by an ailing muscle than dry heat; apply the hot water bottle as needed.

- When the pain has disappeared, resume *very* light weight work for the injured area. If this causes any pain, however, go back to resting this spot and applying the damp hot water bottle as needed. If the light weights are not straining the area, gradually increase the poundage over a period of two to three weeks until you're lifting your normal poundage. Take special care in warming up before your workouts and in keeping the area warm after you've finished exercising.
- Finally, if you ever have any doubt about the seriousness of your injury, do not try to be your own doctor. See a physician if an injury does not respond to your nursing efforts. This could be a sign that you are seriously hurt.

Now that you understand the nature of muscle tissue and body metabolism, as well as how to exercise safely and effectively, you're ready to start working out in earnest. The following chapter contains a glossary of bodybuilding terms to further familiarize you with weight training and fitness.

Chapter 3
Beginning Workout Plan

The following short glossary of the essential bodybuilding/weight training terms is provided to clarify the advice and exercises detailed in this book. Familiarizing yourself with this terminology before your first workout will not only increase your general knowledge of weight training equipment and methods, but you'll also gain a better idea of how to properly execute each exercise as illustrated.

Aerobic Exercise

Extended duration, low intensity exercise relying on consumption and processing of oxygen. Examples of aerobic exercise are jogging, cycling and swimming. By causing your breathing and heart rate to stay elevated for an extended period, aerobic exercise improves and strengthens heart and lung fitness, as well as overall endurance.

Anaerobic Exercise

Short term, high intensity exercise that exceeds the body's aerobic capacity and creates an oxygen debt. Because of its high intensity, anaerobic exercise can only be sustained for brief periods. Weight training, all other resistance exercises and full speed sprinting are prime examples of anaerobic exercise.

Bar

The iron or steel shaft that is the handle of a barbell or dumb-bell. Barbell bars are anywhere from four to seven feet long, while dumb-bell bars are 12 to 16 inches in length. Most bars are one inch in diameter, and are encased in a revolving sleeve.

Barbell

The basic piece of equipment for weight training. A barbell's components are a bar sleeve, collars and plates (see Bar, Sleeve, Collar and Plates). The weight of an adjustable barbell without plates is usually about five pounds per foot of bar length. The weight of a basic barbell unit must be accounted for when you are adding plates to the bar to increase poundage. Barbells in gyms are often fixed with plates of varying poundages welded to the bar. These poundages are marked by numbers painted on the plates of each barbell. Barbells also come in adjustable versions, with assorted weights.

Bodybuilding

An aspect of the sport generally known as weight training, in which the goal is to change the appearance of the physique through a program of weight training and nutrition. For most people, bodybuilding is useful for reducing fatty areas and/or building up thin or weak muscle groups. Bodybuilding is also a competitive sport.

Circuit Training

An advanced method of weight training which develops physical strength and endurance at the same time. Circuit training consists of 10 to 20 exercises using all of the body's major muscle groups. One advances through this circuit in strict order while resting only for a few seconds between sets. Because of its vigorous demands on your muscles and cardiovascular system, circuit training is the quickest route to developing overall strength, endurance and muscle.

Collar

The cylindrical clamp which holds plates in position on a barbell. Inside collars prevent plates from sliding inward and injuring you as you exercise. Outside collars keep the plates from sliding off the end of the bar. Never lift a barbell until you've checked that the collars are firmly fastened.

Definition

The degree to which the muscles are visibly delineated or defined. Muscle definition can be rapidly achieved through programmed weight training and a low-fat diet.

Dumb-bell

A compact version of a barbell, a dumb-bell is lifted in one hand. A classic bodybuilding movement is lifting two equally weighted dumb-bells, one in each hand. Dumb-bells are especially effective for developing muscles in the biceps, triceps, shoulders and forearms. The chest, neck and back are other areas that can be built up through dumb-bell exercises.

Exercise

The actual weight training movement being done, such as a push-up or a seated dumb-bell fly. An exercise is often referred to as a movement.

Flexibility

The degree of suppleness of your muscles and connective tissues. Good flexibility allows one to exercise one's body over a full range of motion.

Form

Form means the proper technique to be used during

the movements of an exercise. One aspect of good weight training form involves inhaling on the relaxation phase and exhaling on the resistance phase. Controlled breathing improves the performance and conditioning of your muscles better than uncontrolled breathing. With the former, you establish a steady and rhythmic oxygen intake which enables the muscles to work to their maximum effort. Good form also requires working the particular muscle group during its range of movement without letting other body parts, such as the back and shoulders, etc, absorb any of the resistance. In any kind of resistance exercise, your first goal should be to execute the movement with proper form. Lifting heavy poundages should only be attempted *after* you have mastered good form.

Hypertrophy
Growth in strength and size of skeletal muscles.

Intensity
The degree of difficulty involved in any given exercise. Intensity can be increased when working with weights by adding poundage, decreasing rest periods between sets, or increasing the number of repetitions done as you exercise. In aerobic exercise, intensity can be increased by simply taking longer strides, strokes, etc, and sustaining these movements at a faster rate.

Lifting Belt
A leather belt, about four to six inches wide at the back. A lifting belt supports and protects the lower back and abdomen from injuries. Many intermediate and advanced back and abdomen exercises require use of a lifting belt for safety's sake. Lifting belts are available at most sporting goods stores and gymnasiums.

Mass
Muscle mass means the size or fulness of muscles.

Muscularity
A synonym for muscle definition.

Poundage
The precise weight of a dumb-bell, barbell or weight machine resistance used in an exercise.

Repetition
Often referred to as a *rep*. A repetition is an individual cycle of an exercise from start to finish and back again. Weight training workouts are composed of multiple repetitions of different exercises.

Resistance
Synonymous with poundage, resistance means the precise weight being used in an exercise.

Rest Interval
The pause between sets of an exercise which allows your muscles to rest; your breathing also gets a chance to return close to normal before beginning the next set of movements. Rest intervals last from 10 to 15 seconds to as much as five minutes. An average rest between sets lasts 60 seconds.

Set
A specific grouping of repetitions, followed by a rest interval and another set. Several sets are usually done for each weight training or resistance exercise in order to build muscle mass and strength.

Sleeve
A hollow metal tube fitted over the bar of a barbell. A sleeve allows a bar to rotate more comfortably in your hands, thus making it easier to lift and hold the barbell. Grooved knurlings are scored into most barbells to aid in maintaining a grip when the hands have become sweaty during a workout.

Spotters
Training partners who stand close by as you train to prevent you from dropping or being pinned under heavy weights, such as a barbell.

Stretching
A type of exercise which develops body flexibility. Stretching involves holding postures which extend certain muscle groups and body parts. Essential for priming the muscles before a workout, stretching relieves muscular tension, stimulates blood circulation and literally warms up your muscles, joints and connective tissues.

Supplements
Concentrated vitamins, minerals or proteins, supplements come in tablet, capsule, powder and liquid form. Food supplements can markedly improve your health by satisfying specific nutritional needs.

Weight
Another word for poundage or resistance. Quite often 'weight' is used to refer to the apparatus (dumb-bell, leg machine, etc) being used in an exercise, as opposed to the exact poundage you happen to be training with.

Weight Training
Various fitness programs involving resistance training exercises and equipment to condition and strengthen the body. The term *weight training* is often used as a synonym for *bodybuilding* or *resistance training exercises*, as these forms of exercise achieve the same results.

Workout
Any exercise session. In this book, however, to work out usually means to perform resistance training exercises.

Warming Up the Right Way

Warm-up exercises are an essential preparation for a workout. Fifteen minutes of warm-ups will increase your heart-rate and pump blood to the muscles where it will soon be needed. Additionally, you can use warm-ups to focus your concentration, further preparing you for a vigorous exercise session.

Rotations

For limbering neck and shoulder muscles, slowly rotate your head around to the right in as wide a circle as possible. Rest 10 seconds and rotate to the left. Repeat. For warming up hands, wrists and forearms, slowly rotate each hand 10 times. For ankles and calves, rotate each foot 10 times.

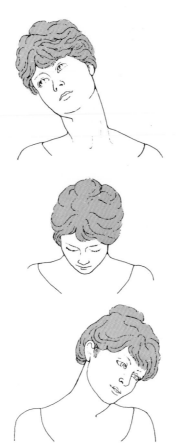

Running in Place

It is important to lift your knees as high up as they can go when doing this. Try to run for at least a minute, increasing your running time each warm-up session.

Scissor Kicks

For buttocks, hips and legs. Lie on your right side with your upper right arm extended and your right hand embracing your head. Plant your left hand on the floor in front; legs should be straight and together. Holding the rest of your body still, raise your left leg straight and as high as you can. Keep your toes flexed backwards as you lift. Lower your leg and repeat 10 times, then switch to other side and lift the right leg.

Side Stretch

When done properly, this is an overall body stretch. Stretch your left hand over your head in an arc and plant your right hand on the floor next to your right knee. Now lift your body up onto your right knee and stretch your left arm over your head. Hold this position for five seconds and feel the resistance. Repeat three times and switch to the other side, bracing your left hand on the floor for support.

Windmills

For shoulders and arms. Stand with your feet 12 inches apart, arms at sides. Make large backward circles with your arms, moving them one after another. Feel the stretch in your arms as you rotate them, and remember to keep your back and waist immobile. Do 10 with each arm: try to work up to being able to do 50 without stopping.

Chair Sit-ups

For abdominal muscles. Lie on your back, hands clasped behind head, heels on a chair. With abdominal muscles tensed, sit up and try to touch your knees with your elbows, exhaling as you bend. Inhale as you slowly lower to original position. If this is too difficult, try extending your arms and touching fingertips to toes instead. Work up to 10 repetitions.

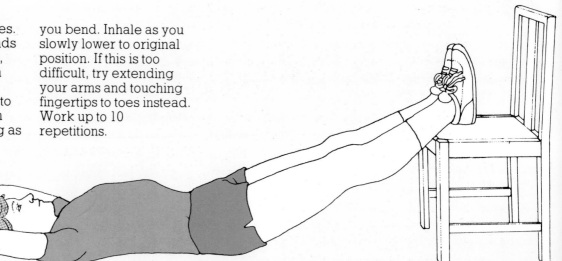

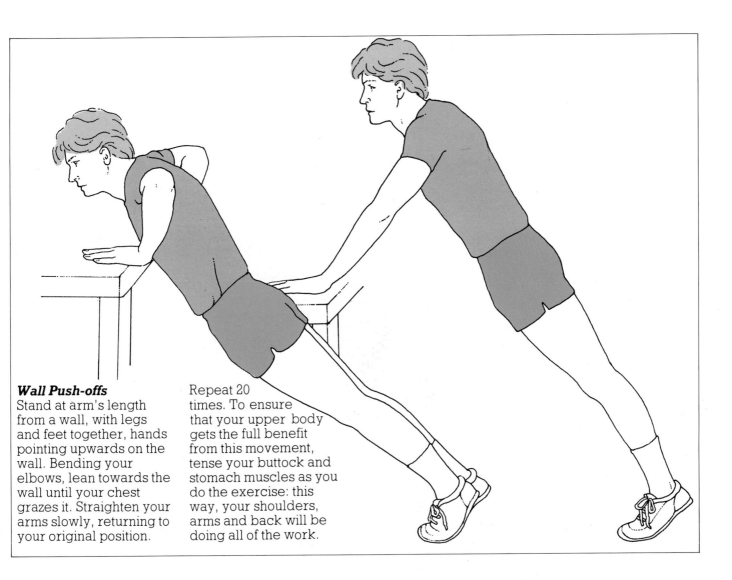

Wall Push-offs
Stand at arm's length from a wall, with legs and feet together, hands pointing upwards on the wall. Bending your elbows, lean towards the wall until your chest grazes it. Straighten your arms slowly, returning to your original position.

Repeat 20 times. To ensure that your upper body gets the full benefit from this movement, tense your buttock and stomach muscles as you do the exercise: this way, your shoulders, arms and back will be doing all of the work.

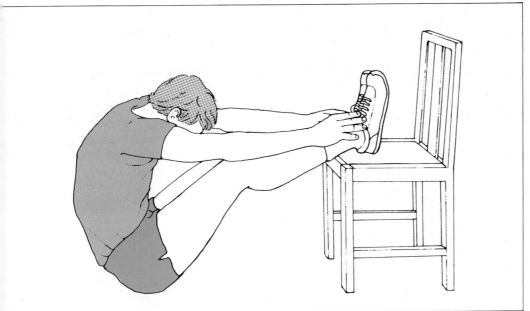

Body Stretch
This is a great way to finish warming up. Begin from a sitting position, with your back straight, left leg extended and right leg bent. Your right foot should be touching your left thigh. Now grasp the ankle of your left leg with both hands and pull your head down to touch your left knee. Stretch the pelvis in this movement by bringing it as near as you can to your thigh. Hold for five seconds. Repeat 10 times and switch to the other leg.

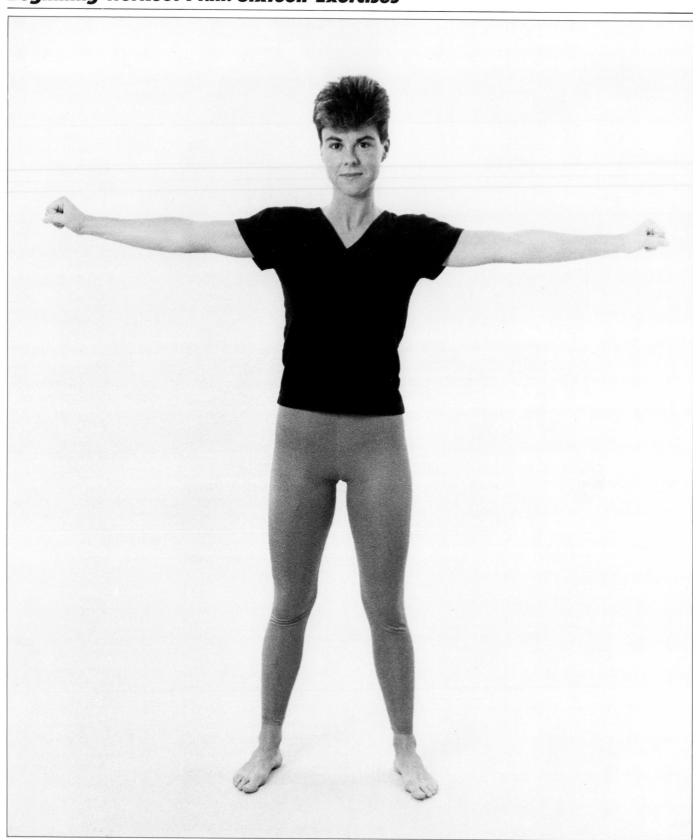

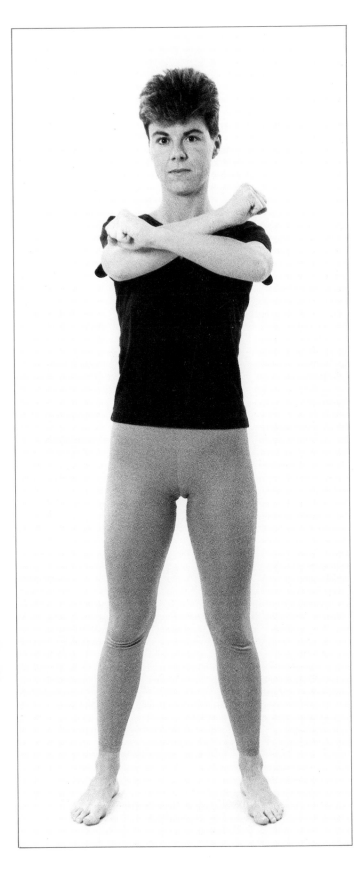

Equipment for these exercises includes a barbell, two dumb-bell bars, and an assortment of plastic-covered weights that fit interchangeably on both the long and short bars. As a beginner, it's preferable that you buy a weight set that includes 2½ lb plates, since the smaller plates allow you to increase poundage more gradually as you get in shape. With 2½ lb plates, for example, you can add 5 lbs to the bar (one 2½ lb plate on each end), while with 5 lb plates, you can only add 10 lbs (one 5 lb plate on each end) at a time. Increasing poundage in 10 lb weights is usually too strenuous for those who are new to weight training. Play it safe and use 5 lb dumb-bells at the start; barbell poundage should also be as light as possible.

Please note, however, that half of these Beginning exercises require only your own weight — or books and furniture — as resistance equipment. These exercises can be easily integrated into your daily schedule; you can do them in an office or hotel room as a substitute for your regular workout. No matter where or when you exercise, though, it's a good idea to perform the exercises in the order in which they are given here. This is because the plan works the larger muscle areas first, in an order that ensures that your body gets an optimum workout without tiring in the middle of the session.

One final word of advice: do not be discouraged if initially you fail to complete all the repetitions specified for an exercise. As a beginner, this is to be expected. Just try to concentrate on completing each movement with proper form and maximum effort, and strength will develop in a matter of weeks.

Chest Exercises

1. Standing Cross-arm Flies

(One set, 20 repetitions) Stand with your feet shoulder-width apart; arms held straight at the sides. Slowly, feeling the pull in the chest, cross your arms, left over right, pulling each across your chest as far as it will stretch. Then bring them back to starting position for one repetition. On the next rep, cross your right arm over your left, and continue to alternate arms throughout the set.

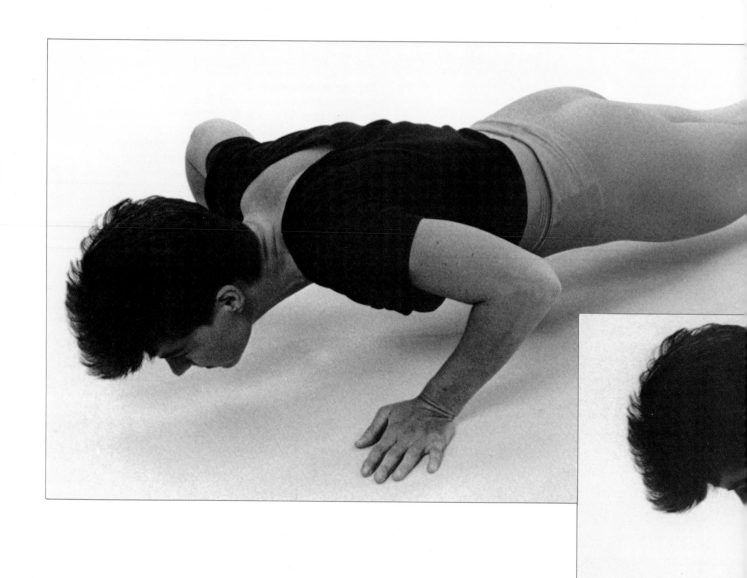

2. Push-ups

(One set, 10 repetitions) Lying almost on your stomach, place your hands palms down on the floor on a level with your chest. Your hands should be a little more than shoulder-width apart. Now, keeping your head down and your back straight, slowly push up until your arms are fully extended.

Slowly lower yourself so that your chest brushes the floor for one repetition. Remember to inhale as you lower yourself; exhale as you push up. Exhaling on the resistance phase of an exercise always gives you added energy to complete the repetition. Try to work up to 20 repetitions.

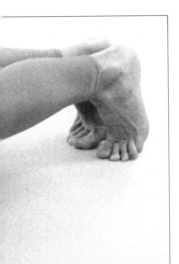

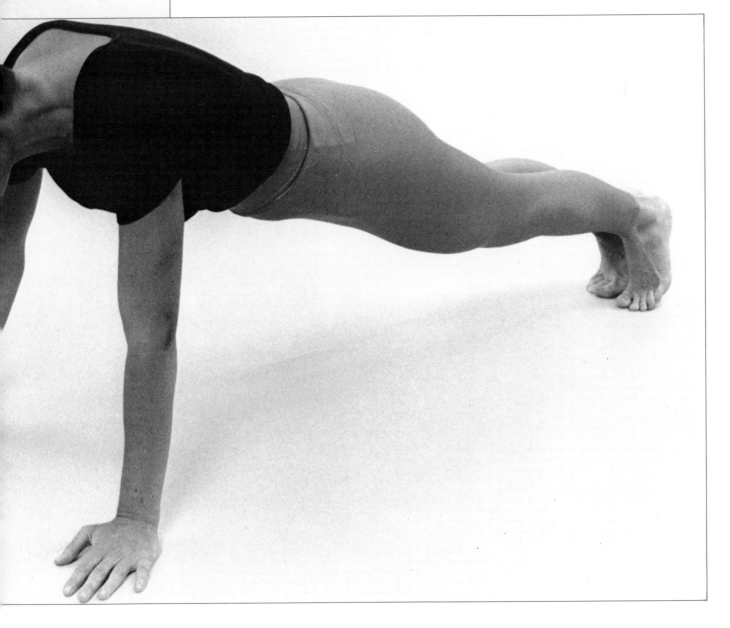

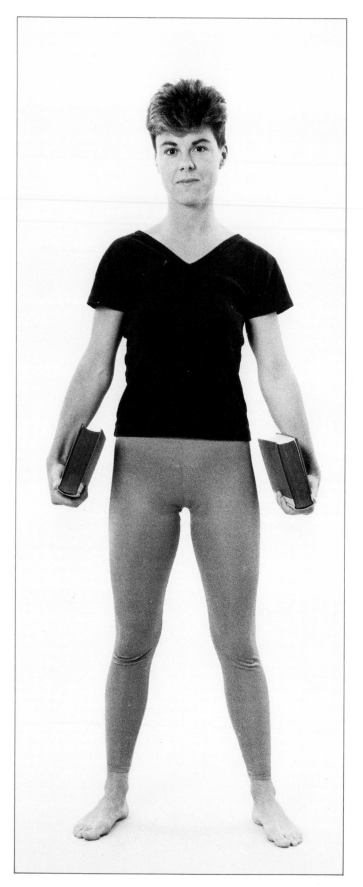

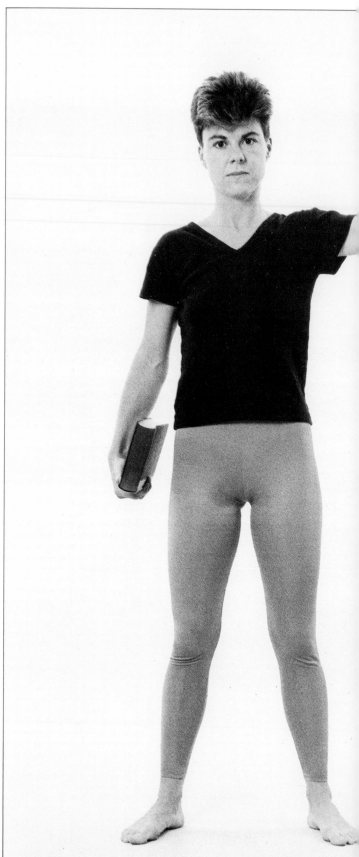

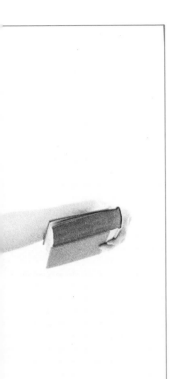

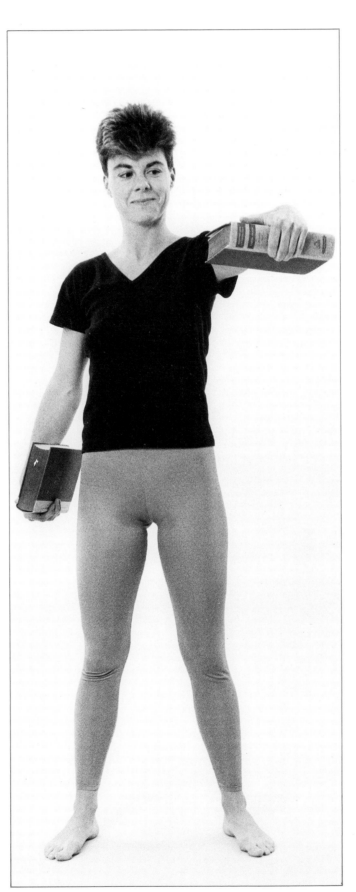

Shoulder Exercises

1. Standing Front and Lateral Flies

(One set, 20 repetitions with each arm) Standing up straight, take two books of equal weight; grasp one in each hand, at hip level. Lift your left arm out to the side, to shoulder level, keeping the arm straight; now lower it to your hip again and lift it up in front of you to shoulder level. Lower it again for one repetition. Alternate left and right arms for 20 repetitions with each. Concentrate on making your shoulder do the pulling as you lift the books.

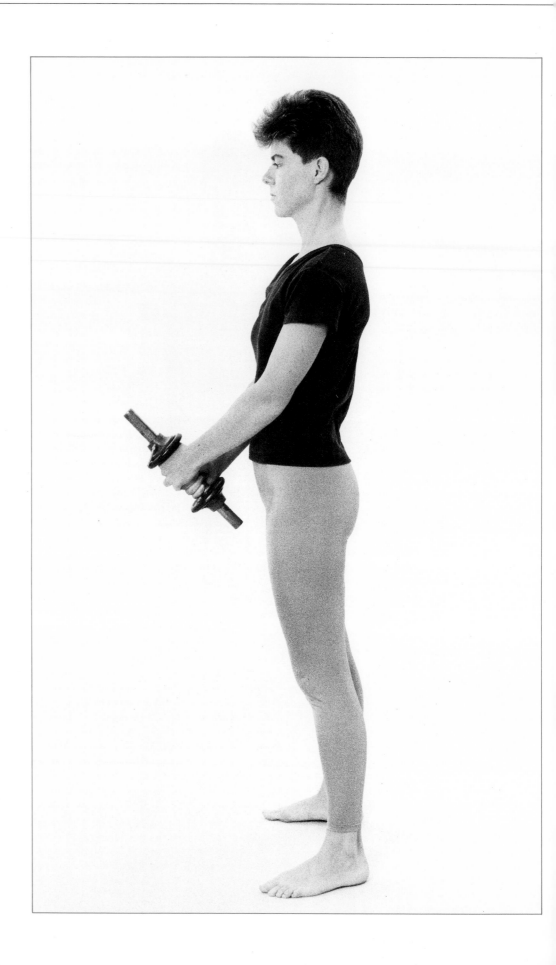

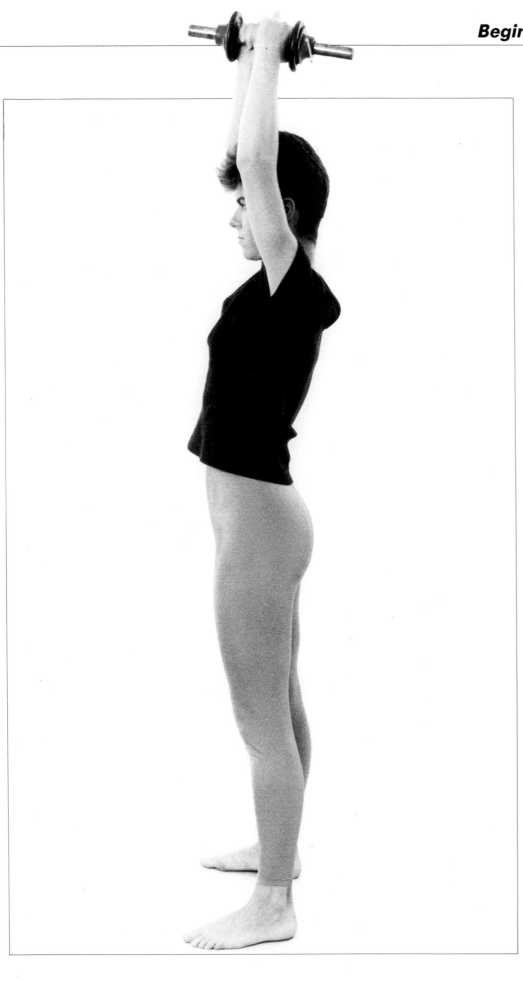

2. Front Dumb-bell Raises

(One set, 15 repetitions) Stand with your feet about 1½ ft apart, holding a dumb-bell with both hands in front of your legs. Keep your back straight and immobile as you raise the dumb-bell directly over your head and then lower it slowly in one smooth motion.

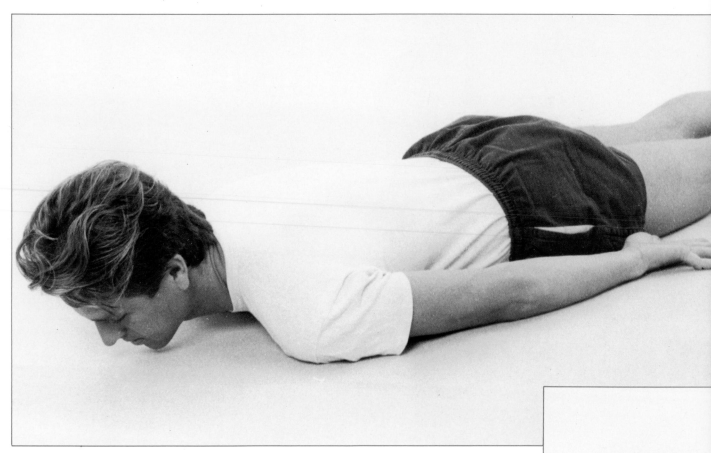

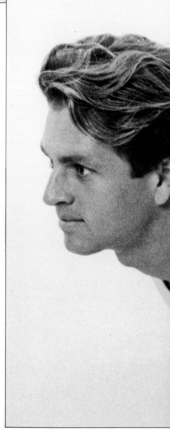

Back Exercises

1. Lower Back Extensions

(One set, 15 repetitions) Lie on your stomach and chest with your head off the floor; your arms lying behind you and to the sides. Now curl your legs and upper body up towards each other as far as they stretch. Only your stomach and hips should remain on the floor as you hold this 'arc' position for one repetition. (This exercise also happens to be good for toning the buttocks.)

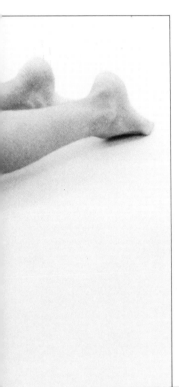

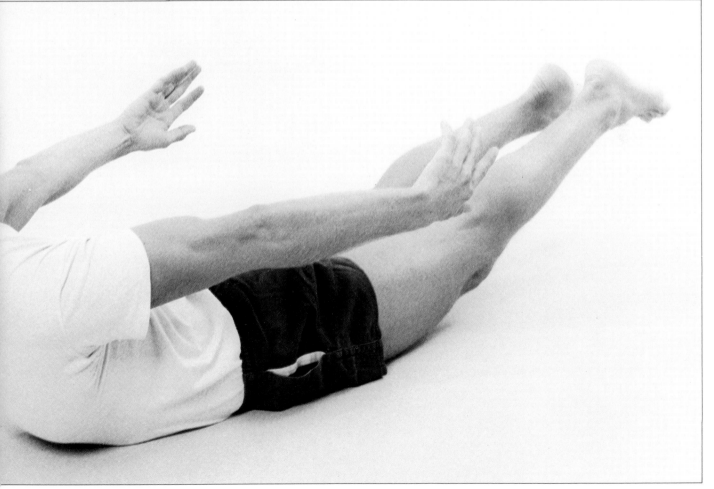

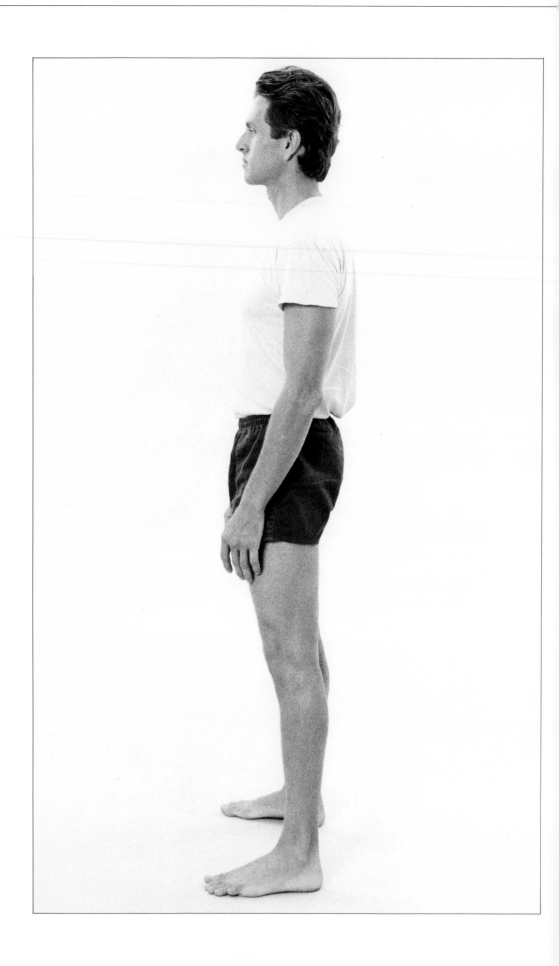

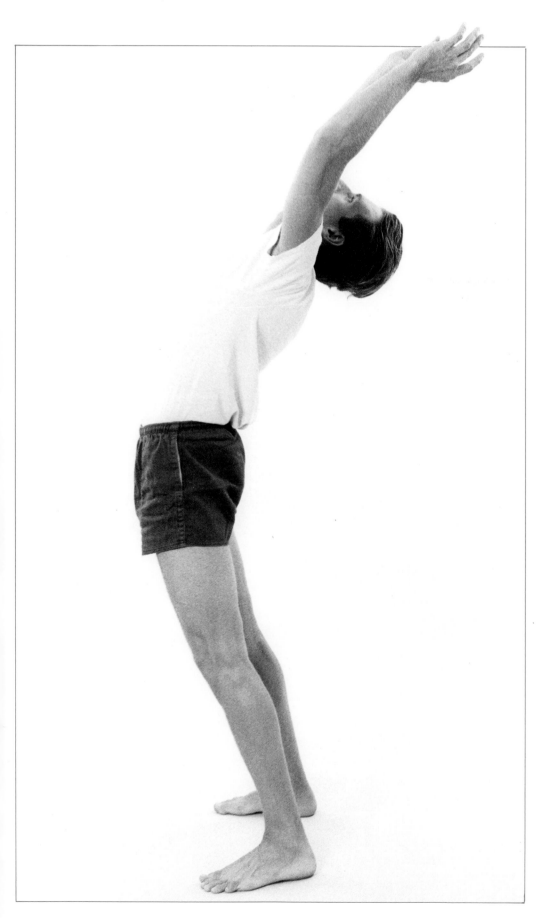

2. Back Bends

(One set, 10 repetitions) Stand up straight, with arms at sides. Now bend backwards as far as you can, letting your arms stretch upwards in front of your chest. Using only your abdominal muscles, *slowly pull* yourself upright. A slight burning sensation in the abdominal muscles indicates that you are doing the exercise correctly.

Biceps Exercises

1. Seated Dumb-bell Biceps Curls

(One set, 10 repetitions) Do this exercise seated in a chair, with your back straight, arms held out slightly at the sides. Your hands hold the dumb-bells below your hips with palms facing upwards. Keeping the backs of your arms taut and your back immobile, slowly curl both dumb-bells up toward your shoulders. Raise the dumb-bells only as high as the point where you can still feel tension in the front of your upper arms — never pull them all the way up to your shoulders. Now, lower them slowly, maintaining the tension, for one repetition.

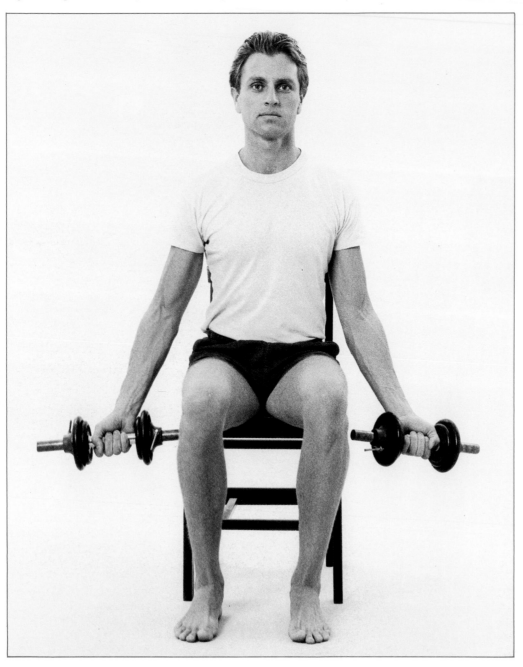

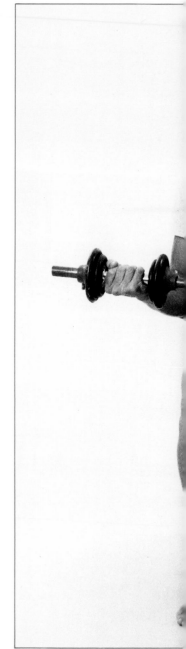

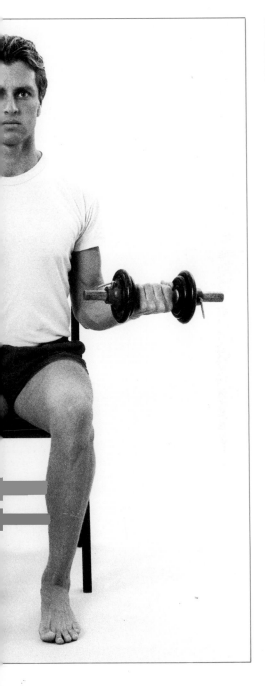

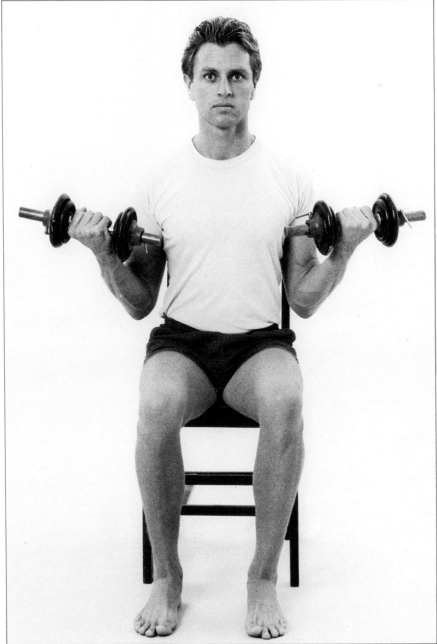

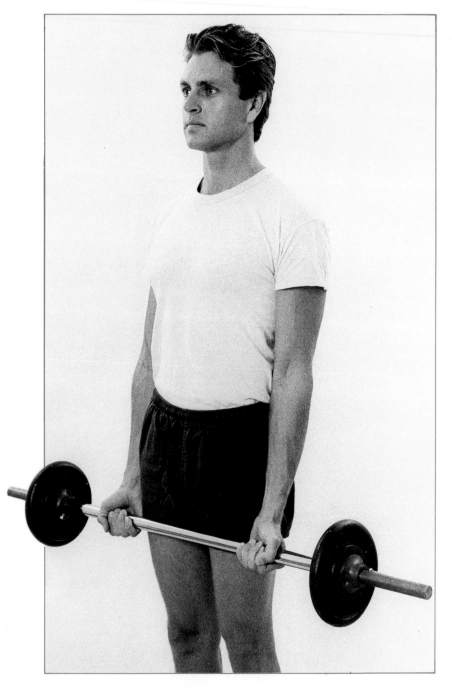
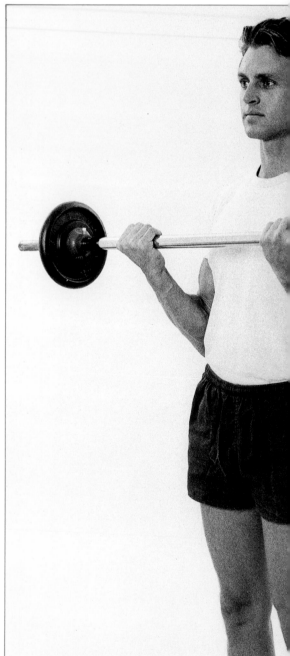

2. Barbell Curls

(One set, 10 repetitions) Take a shoulder-width undergrip (palms facing up) on a barbell. Stand erect and straighten your arms, pressing your upper arms against the sides of your torso. Keeping your upper arms motionless, use only your biceps' strength to raise the barbell from the front of your thighs to a point beneath your chin where you can still feel tension in the biceps. Slowly lower the barbell, again keeping the tension in your biceps, for one repetition.

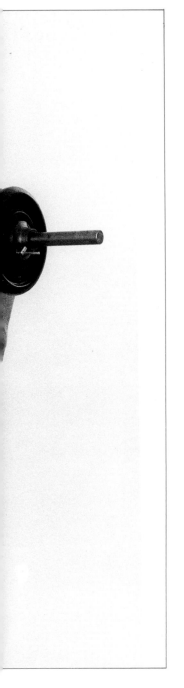

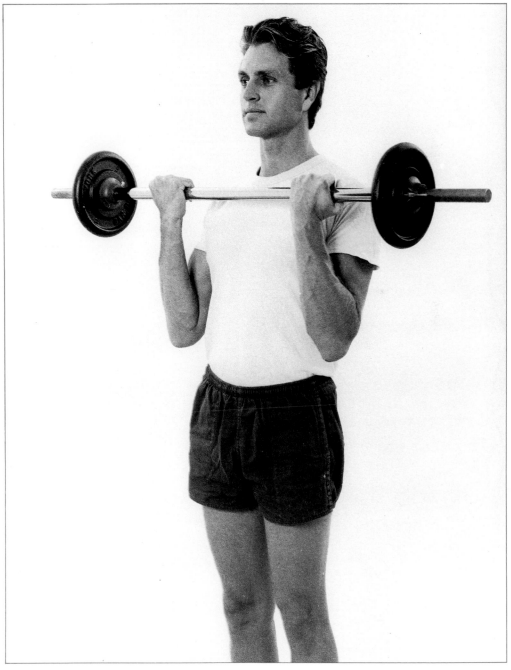

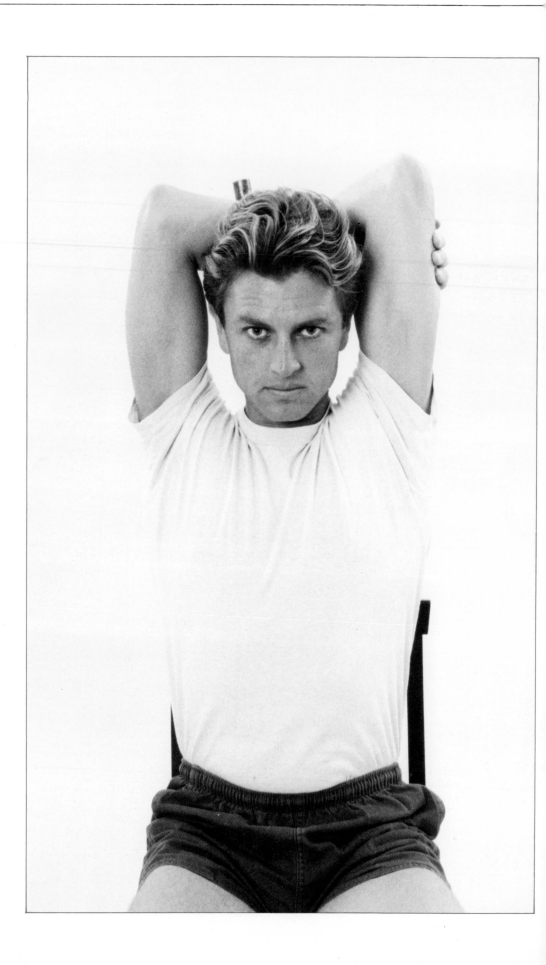

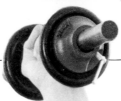

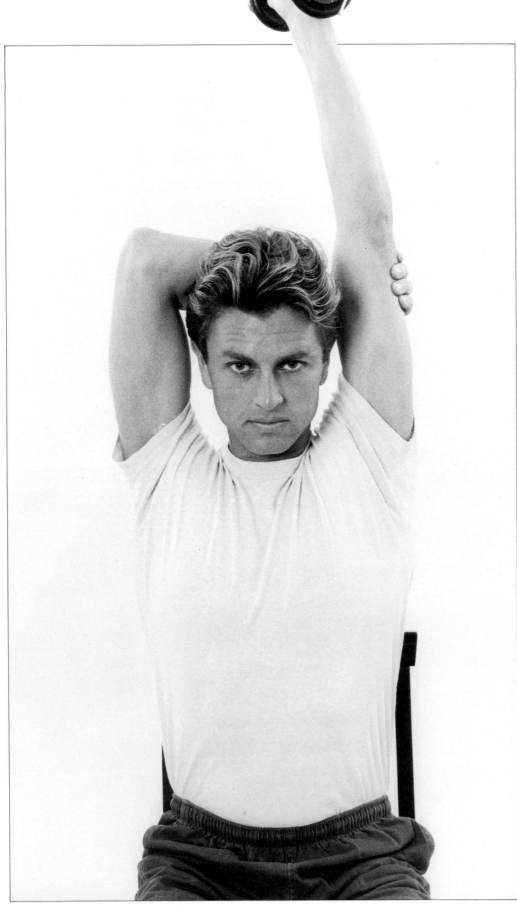

Triceps Exercises

1. One Arm Triceps Press

(One set, five reps with each arm)
Sitting in a chair, grasp a dumb-bell at one end in your left hand behind your shoulders. Your right elbow should be pointing up towards the ceiling. Bending your right arm at the elbow, cross it behind your head to grip the outside of your upper left arm. Now lower the weight as far as you can, feeling the muscle work with your right hand. Next, slowly raise the weight to an almost full extension of your arm. Lower again to starting position. Do five reps and switch to the left arm for five more.

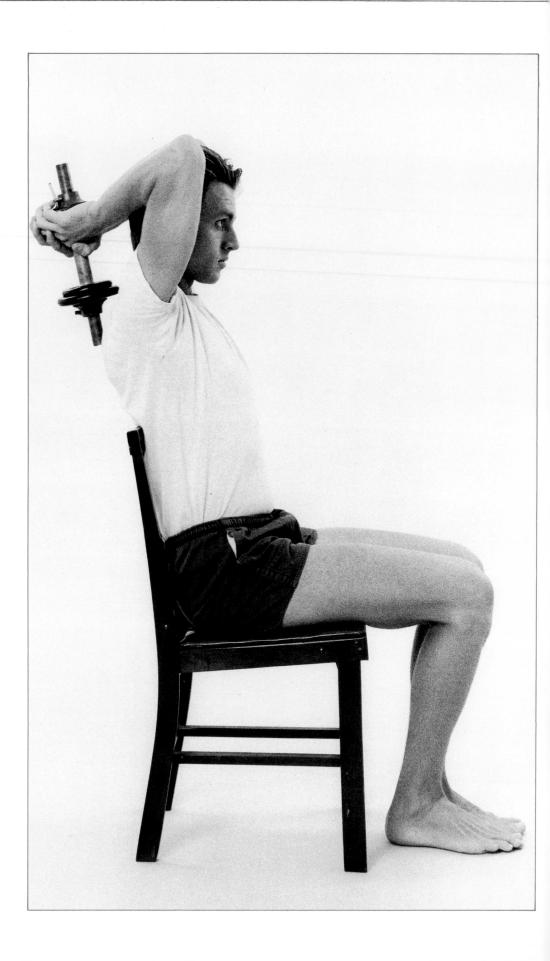

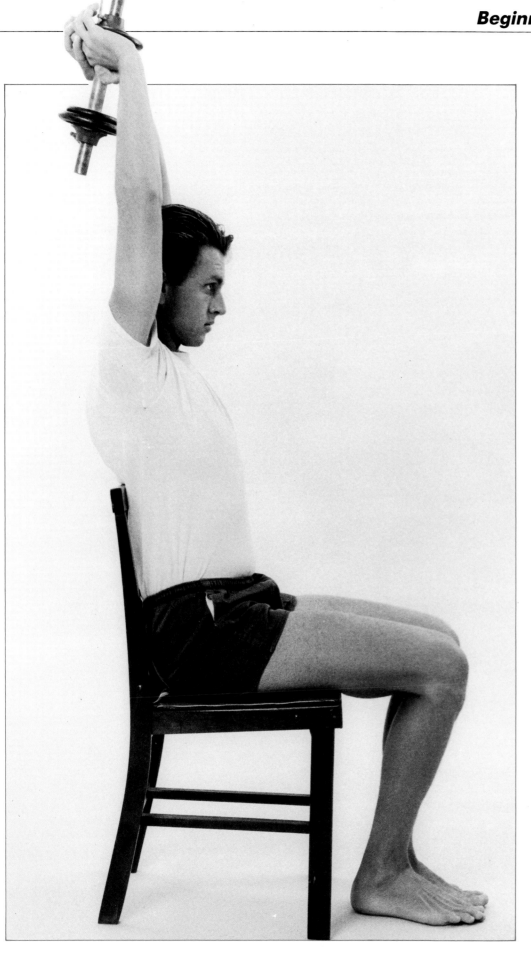

2. Seated Dumb-bell Triceps Press

(One set, 10 repetitions) Sitting up straight in a chair, hold a dumb-bell behind your head in both hands as shown. Your elbows should point towards the ceiling; upper arms should stay immobile. Now, smoothly raise the dumb-bell overhead for one repetition.

Leg Exercises

1. Alternating Standing Kickbacks

(One set, 10 repetitions with each leg)
Stand 2½ to 3ft away from a chair with feet slightly parted. Bend over and place your hands on the chair for support; your head should be higher than your hips. Now raise one leg and kick back as pictured, feeling the muscles in the lower back, buttocks and legs as they stretch. Lower leg and switch to the other. Alternate for 10 reps with each leg.

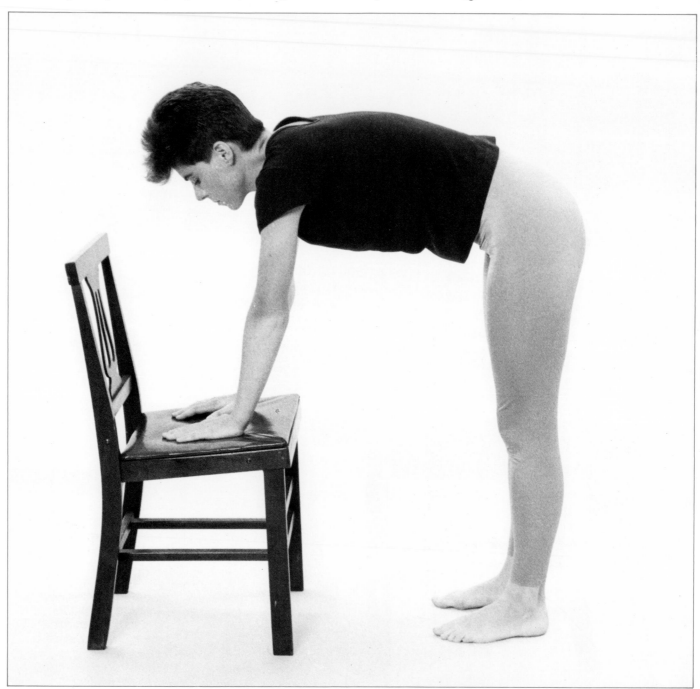

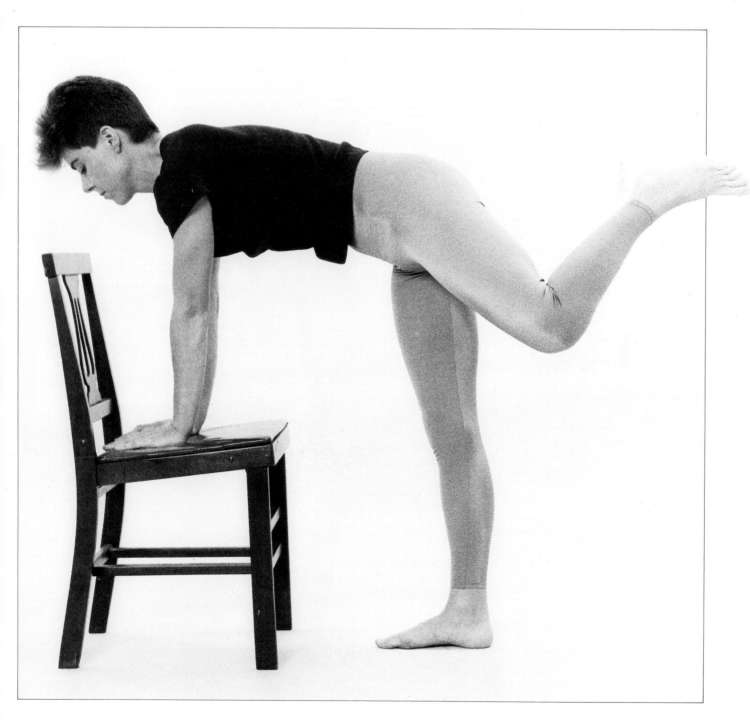

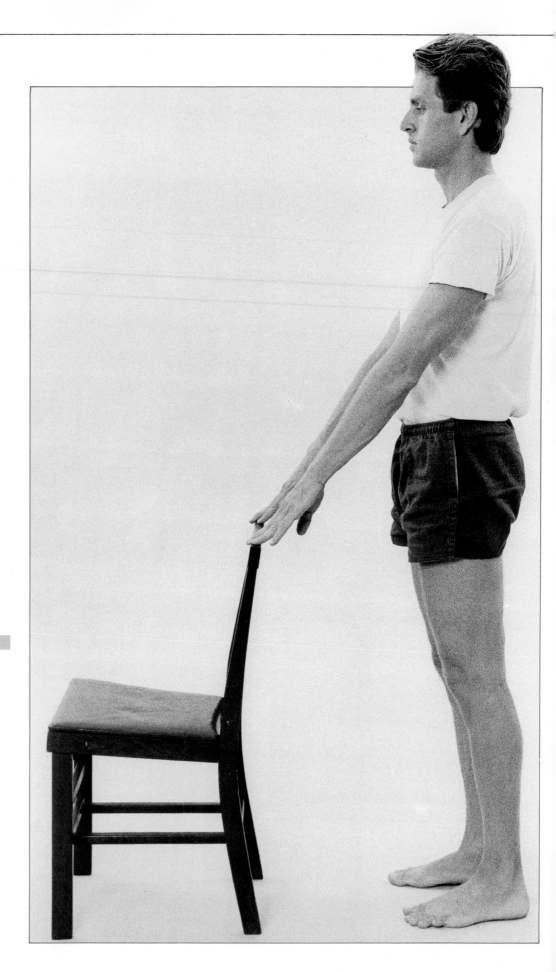

2. Deep Knee Bends

(One set, 20 repetitions)
Hold onto a chair that is
below waist height to
keep your balance
during this exercise.
Your feet should be a
few inches apart. Keep
your back perfectly
straight as you slowly
lower yourself and rise
up to complete each
repetition. Let your
quadriceps do all the
work: they may feel
slightly strained at first,
but you should be able
to work up to 40
repetitions within a few
weeks.

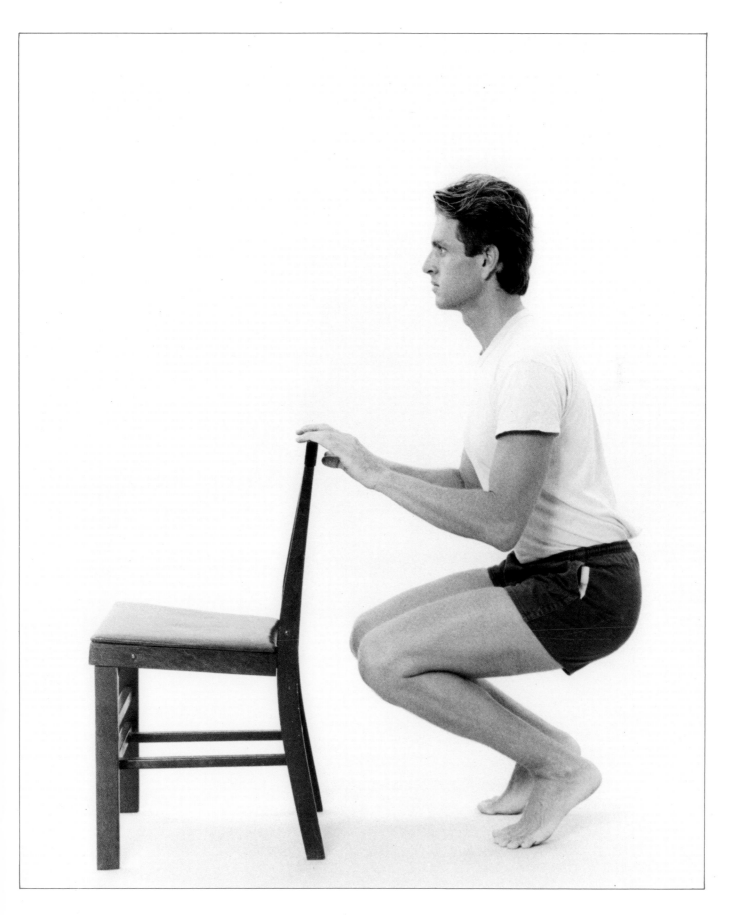

Calf Exercises

1. Leg Curls With Dumb-bells

(One set, eight repetitions with each leg)
To do this you need either a belt or a strap. Put one end of the strap around the dumb-bell and the other end around the ankle of your right leg. Grasping the back of a chair for support, bend at the waist and try to keep your back flat. Lift your right leg behind you so that the dumb-bell is slightly above the floor; do not let it touch the floor during the exercise. Next, raise your heel up towards your buttocks as far as it will go. Lower steadily for one repetition. Remember to maintain proper breathing form as you go — it will help you exert your muscles to their maximum strength.

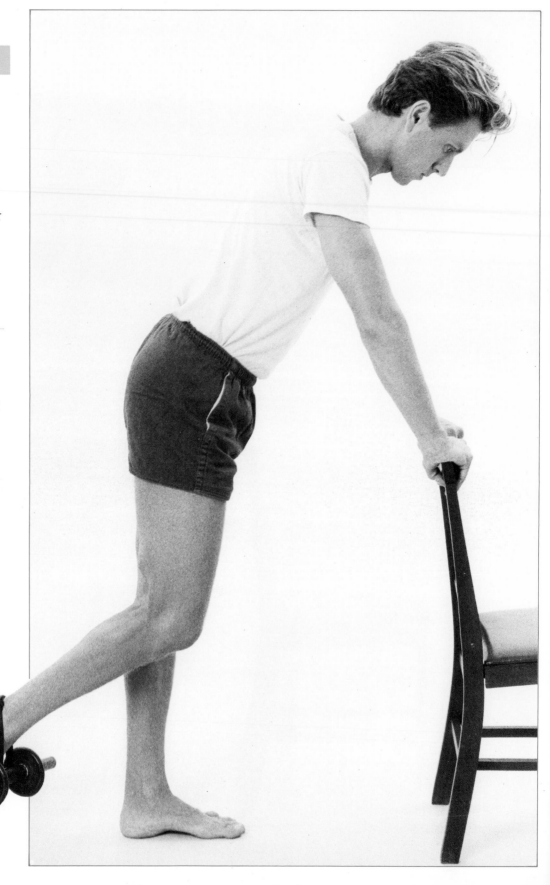

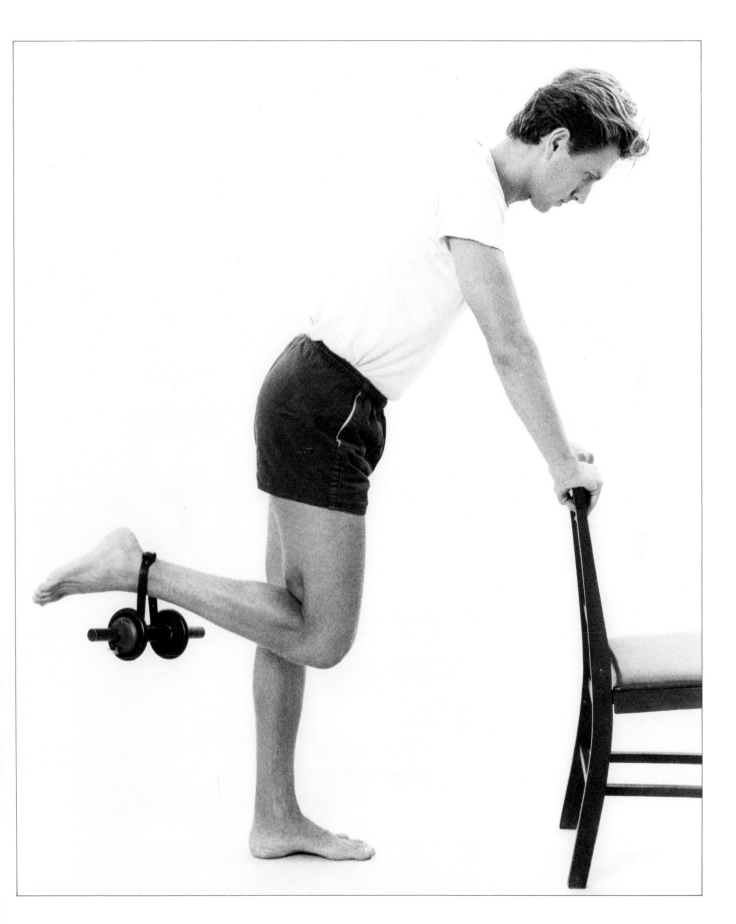

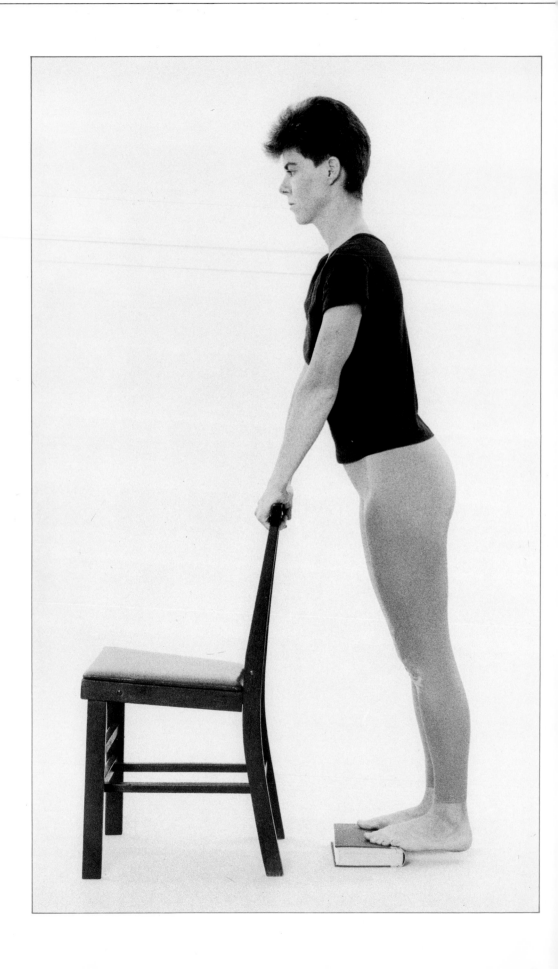

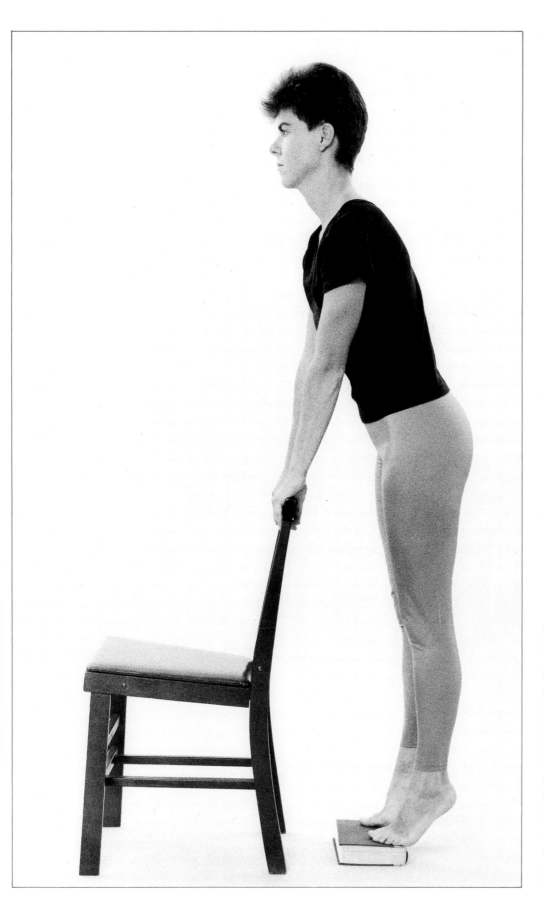

2. Calf Raises

(One set, 10 repetitions)
Stand on top of a thick
book with feet an inch or
two apart — your heels
should hang over the
edge. Lightly grasping
the back of a chair for
support, use your calf
muscles to raise yourself
up on your toes. Hold for
three seconds and
slowly lower for one
repetition. Try to work
up to 20 reps within two
weeks. Besides being an
excellent calf-toner, this
exercise will also
improve your balance.

Abdominal Exercises

1. Waist Crunch

(One set, 10 repetitions) This is especially beneficial for the lower abdominal muscles. Lie on your back with your hands tucked under your hips. Lift your legs about 6 ins off the floor. Bring your knees in to your chest as close as you can. Then stretch your legs out straight again for one repetition. Your legs and feet should stay *above* the floor throughout the set.

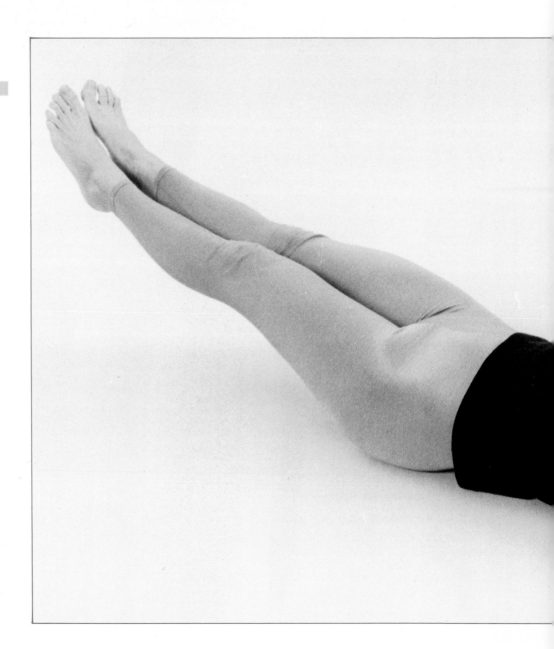

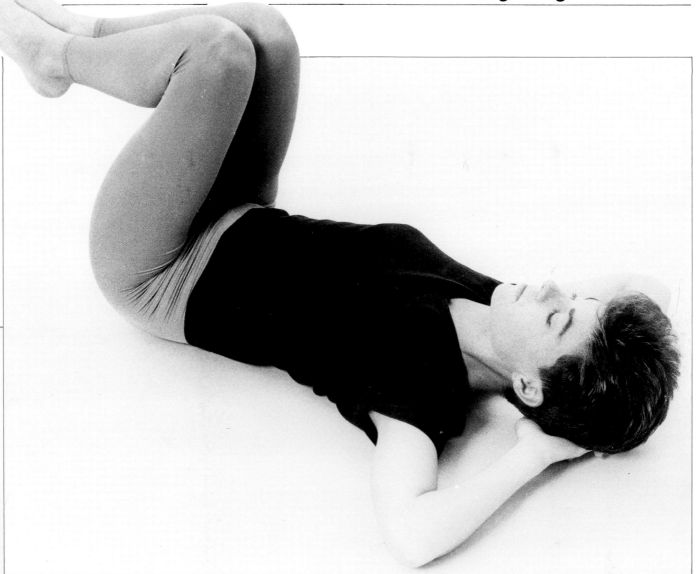

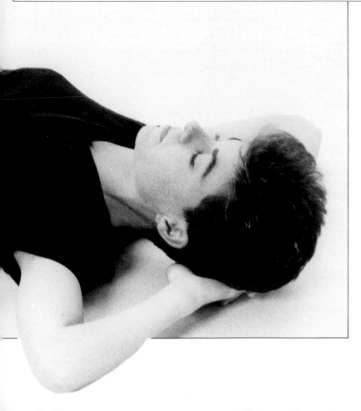

2. Bent Leg Sit-ups

(One set, 10 repetitions) Lie on your back with legs about shoulder-width apart, or wider, as you may have difficulty doing this exercise at first. Clasping your hands behind your head, slowly curl your body up so that your elbows touch your knees. Use only your stomach muscles to raise yourself; keep your back as straight as you can while smoothly lowering your body back to starting position. Pay attention to your breathing form as you go. Try to increase the number of repetitions each time you work out — you should be able to do a set of 20 repetitions after three weeks.

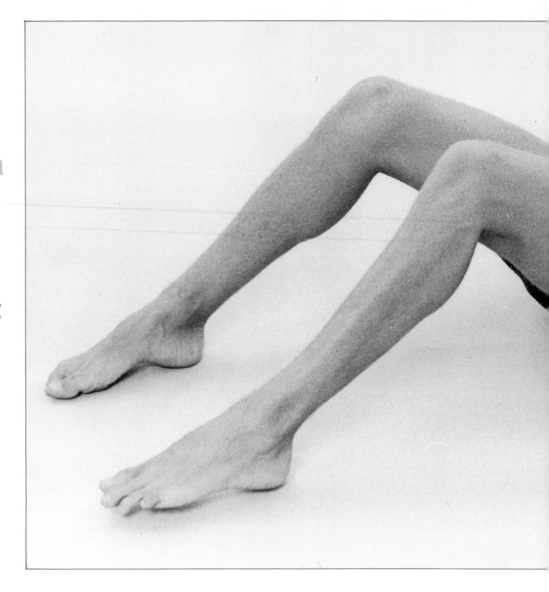

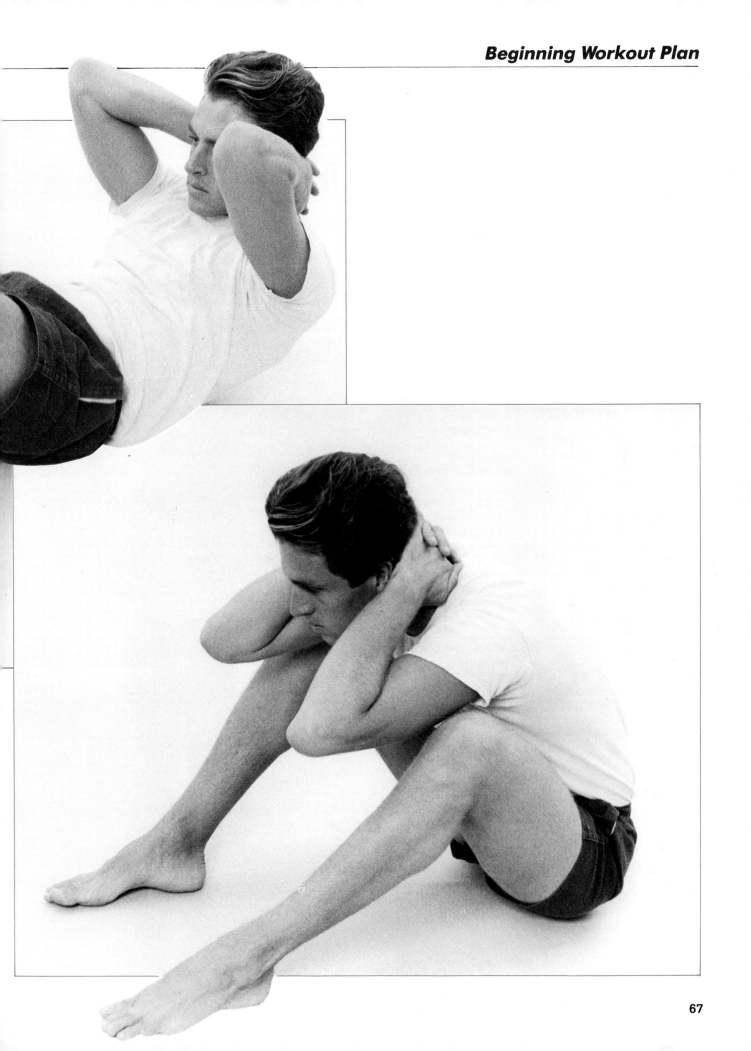

Chapter 4

Intermediate Workout Plan

Warming Up

Review Chapter 3's warm-up exercises as well as the Beginning Workout Plan. Select exercises from both sections that involve each muscular group. Spend 15 minutes or more warming up, and concentrate on maintaining proper form at all times.

Chest Exercises

1. Standing Cross Arm Flies With Dumb-bells

(One Set, 10 repetitions) Stand with feet shoulder-width apart, arms held out at sides, a dumb-bell in each hand. (NB: 5 lb dumb-bells are recommended here, or, perhaps 8 lb dumb-bells.) Increase poundage *only* when you can complete 10 reps without feeling resistance. Now, slowly cross your arms, left over right, pulling each across your chest as far as you can go. Then slowly return to starting position for one repetition.

2. Push-ups

(Two sets, 10 repetitions for each set)
This is a variation of Chest Exercise 2 in the Beginning Workout Plan. Do 10 push-ups, then stand up and walk around for a minute while your breathing returns to normal. Then do another 10.

Shoulder Exercises

1. Standing Dumb-bell Presses

(One set, 15 repetitions) Stand with feet 12 to 18 ins apart, holding the two dumb-bells at shoulder-level. With back straight, press the dumb-bell in your right hand to an *almost* full extension of the arm. Lower the dumb-bell slowly and do 15 repetitions with each arm.

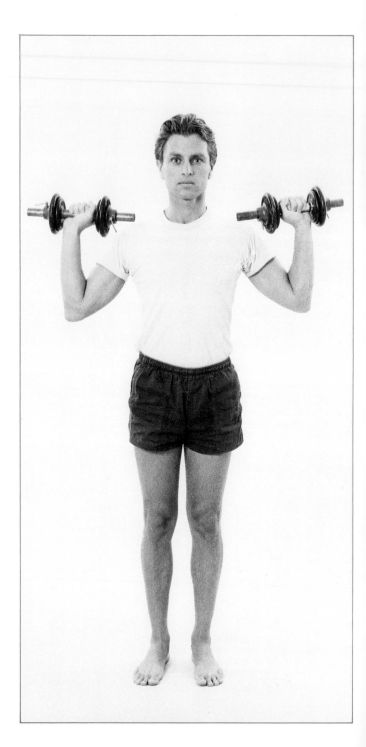

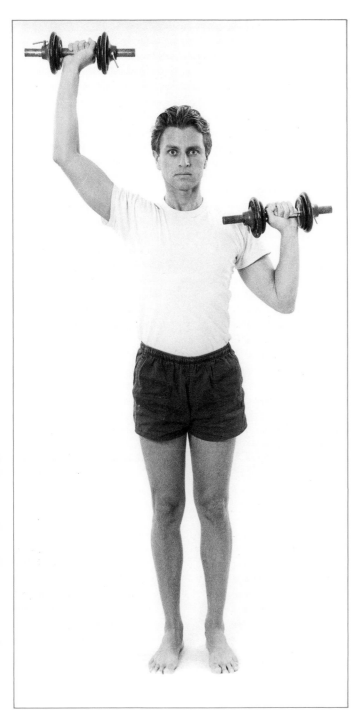
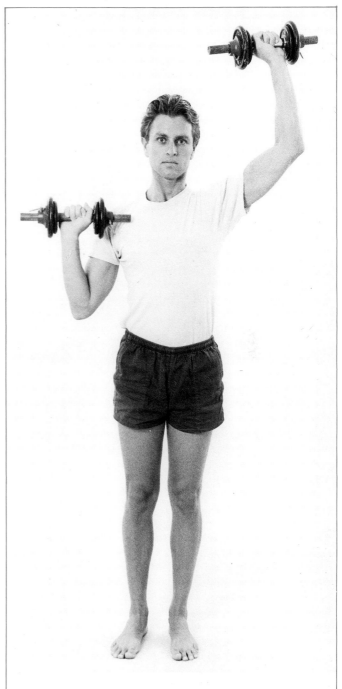

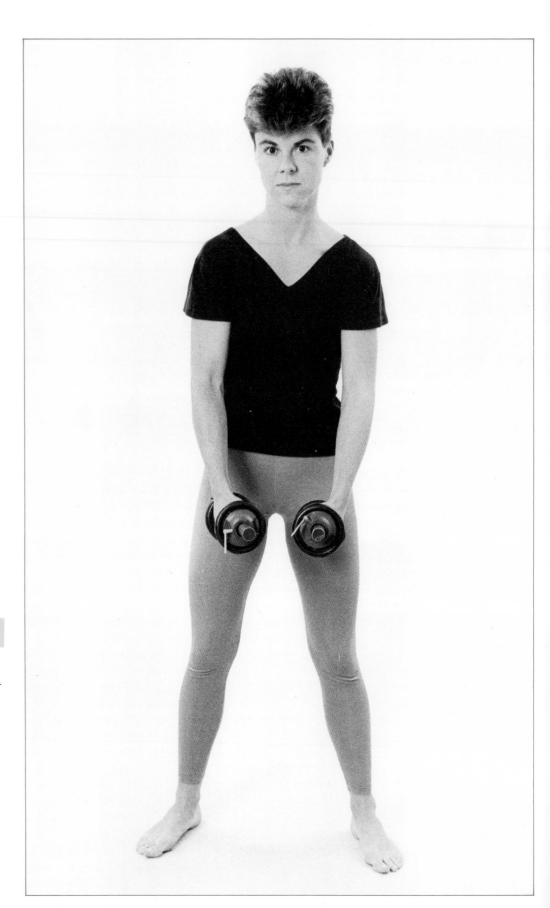

2. Standing Dumb-bell Flies

(One set, 15 repetitions) Stand with feet shoulder-width apart, holding the two dumb-bells in front of your hips, palms facing each other, with your arms semi-bent at the elbow, and leaning slightly forward at the waist. Now lift your arms up in front of your body, bringing dumb-bells up to head level. Then lower them steadily to original position for one repetition.

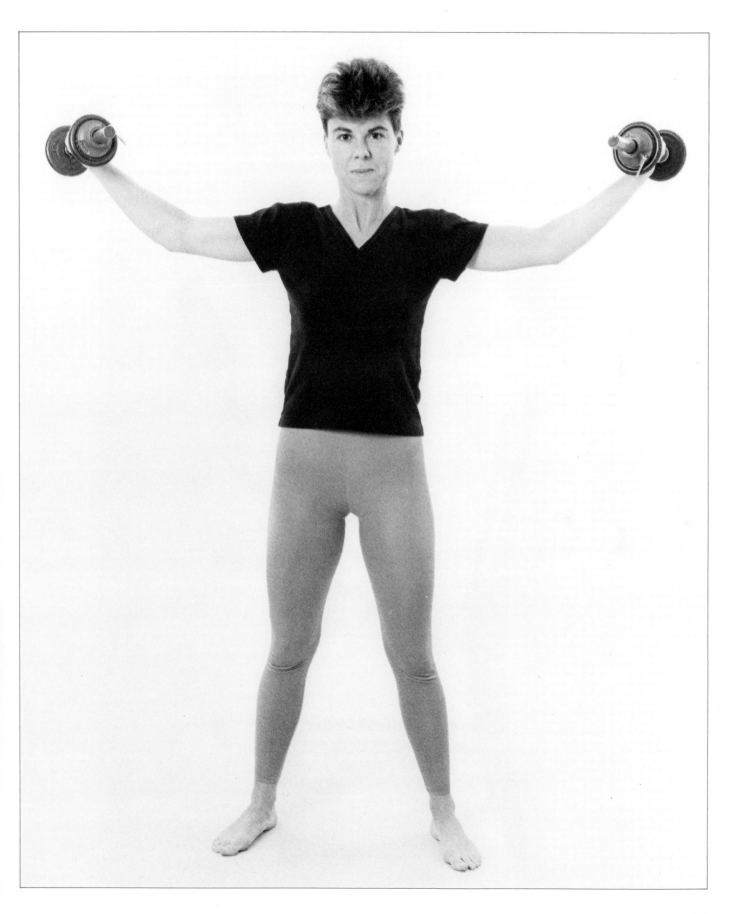

Back Exercises

1. Alternating Dumb-bell Rows

(One set, 15 repetitions with each arm)
Stand with left leg on the floor; your right leg resting on a chair at about knee level. Place your right arm on the chair for support; hold the dumb-bell in your left hand. Your left arm should be fully extended downwards. (Relax both arms to allow your back muscles to lift the weight.) Now slowly raise the dumb-bell to your chest; then lower it to original position for one rep. Do 15 reps with left arm, then 15 with right arm.

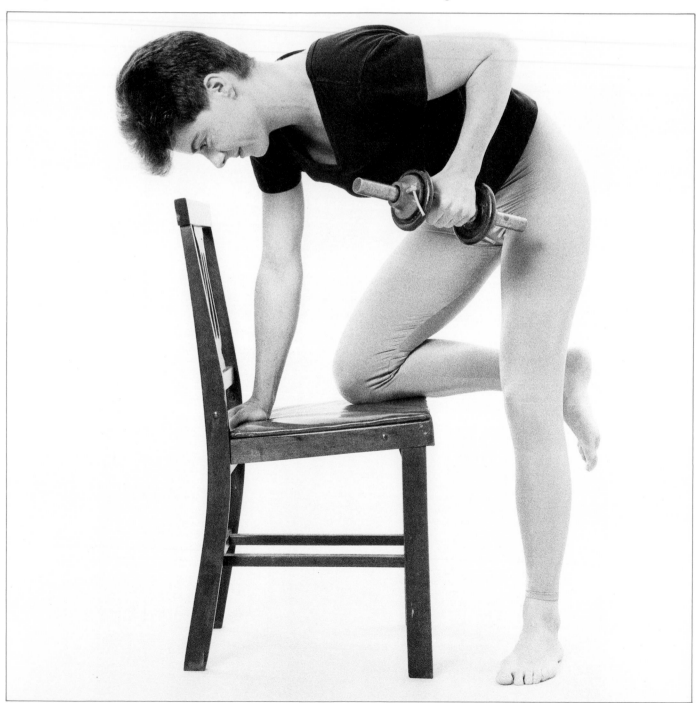

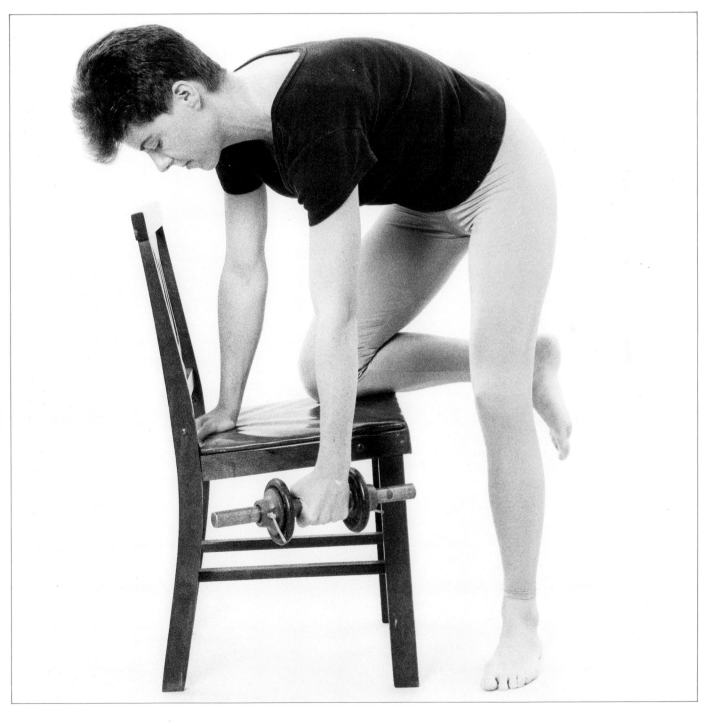

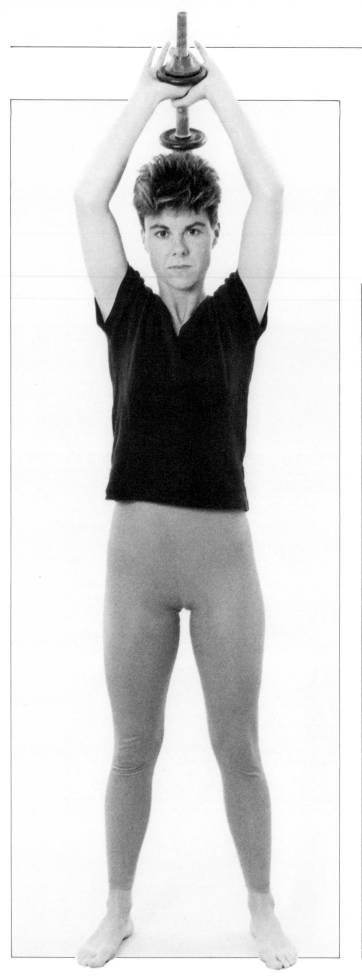

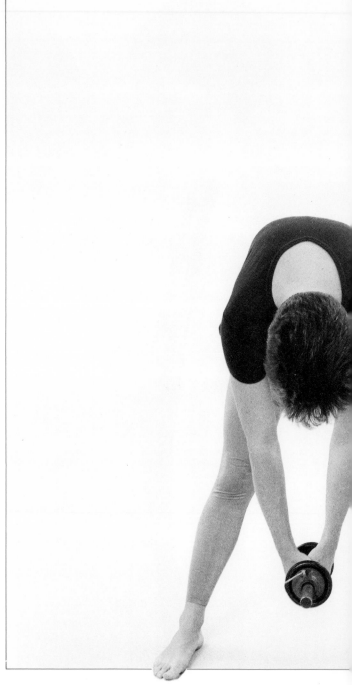

2. Dumb-bell Swings

(One set, 15 repetitions) Space your feet a little wider than shoulder-width. Hold one dumb-bell in both hands above your head. Bend forward at the waist and swing your arms down between your legs, then come up again with arms extended in front of you. Try not to bend your arms too much at the elbows. Use only your lower back to lift your torso and arms back upright for one repetition. This exercise must be done at a slow, steady speed for maximum benefit, so take care to do it properly.

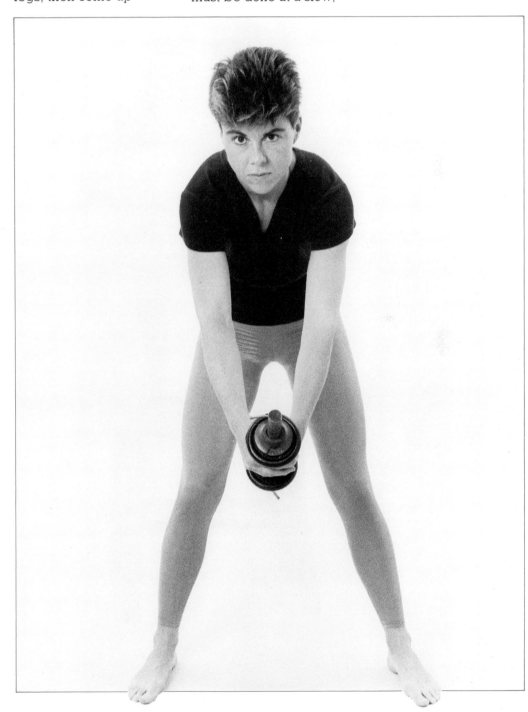

Biceps Exercises

(Not illustrated)

1. Seated Dumb-bell Biceps Curls

(Two sets, 10 repetitions each set)
This is a variation on Biceps Exercise 1 in the Beginning Workout. Do the exercise as instructed there, and rest for three minutes after you've completed 10 reps. Then do 10 more.

2. Barbell Curls

(Two sets, 10 repetitions each set)
This is a variation on Biceps Exercise 2 in the Beginning Workout Plan; you can further increase the intensity of this exercise by adding poundage to the barbell. Do 10 reps and then rest for three minutes, walking about or stretching while your breathing slows back down to normal. Do another set of 10 and rest a few minutes before going on to the next exercise.

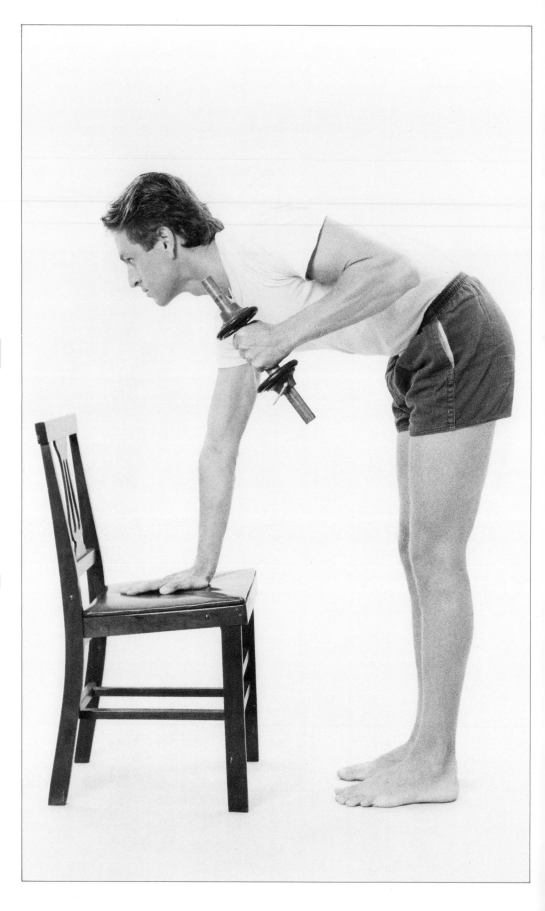

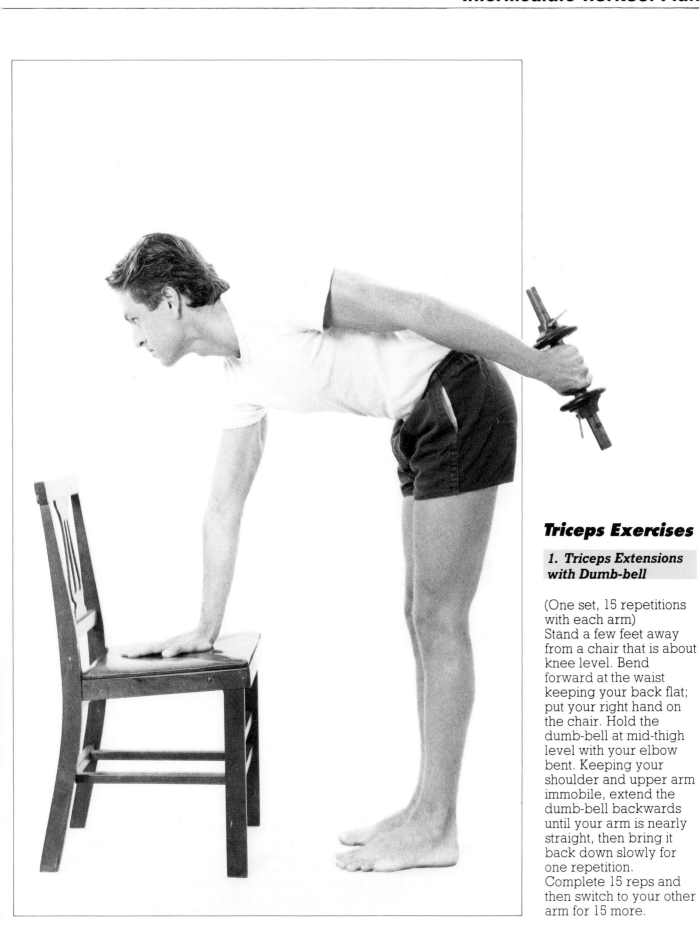

Triceps Exercises

1. Triceps Extensions with Dumb-bell

(One set, 15 repetitions with each arm)
Stand a few feet away from a chair that is about knee level. Bend forward at the waist keeping your back flat; put your right hand on the chair. Hold the dumb-bell at mid-thigh level with your elbow bent. Keeping your shoulder and upper arm immobile, extend the dumb-bell backwards until your arm is nearly straight, then bring it back down slowly for one repetition. Complete 15 reps and then switch to your other arm for 15 more.

2. Seated One Arm Triceps Press

(Two sets, 10 repetitions with each arm)
Hold two dumb-bells at shoulder height. Slowly raise one upwards, using only the muscle in the back of your upper arm. Steadily lower to starting position. Do 10 reps with each arm.

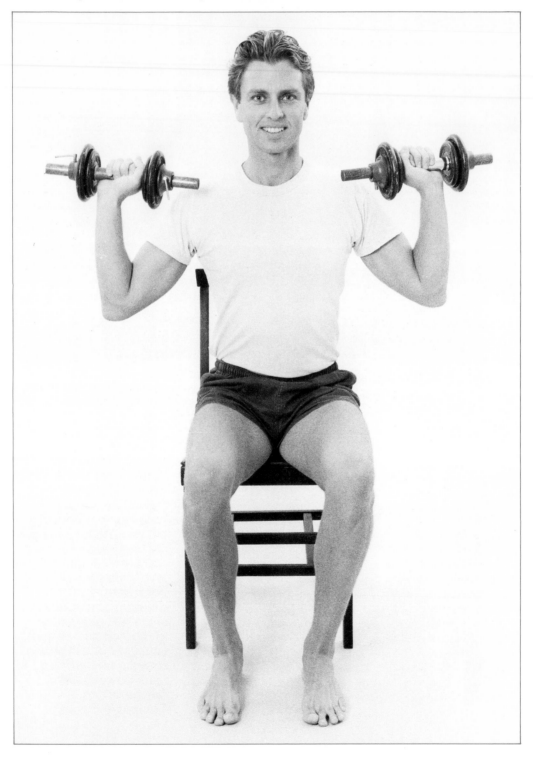

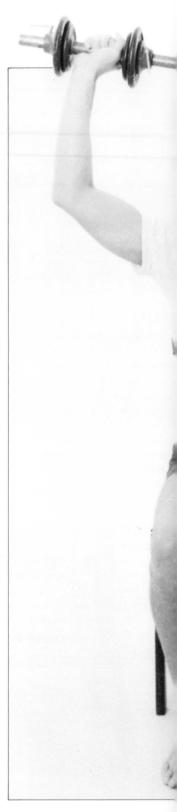

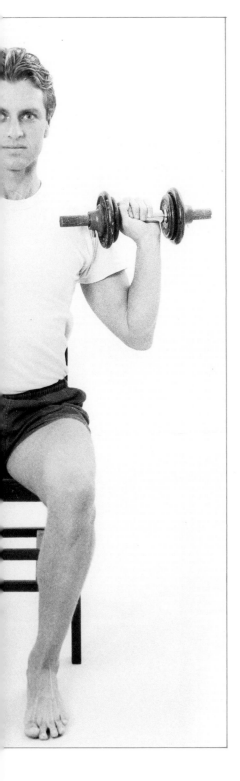

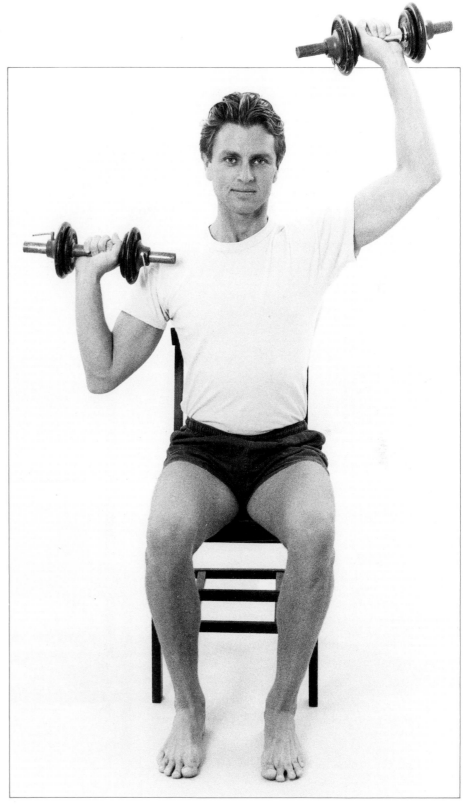

Leg Exercises

1. Deep Knee Bends

(One set, 40 repetitions)
A variation on Leg
Exercise 2. Maintain
proper breathing form
as you complete a set of
40 reps; feel the muscles
in the front of your thighs
as you lower and raise
yourself, keeping your
back straight as you go.

2. Standing Leg Kicks

(Two sets, 15 repetitions
with each leg)
Stand behind a chair
and hold onto it for
balance. Keeping your
hips straight, raise your
right leg out to the side
as high as it will go, then
slowly lower it, feeling
the resistance. Do 15
reps with that leg and
then switch to the left.
Take a one minute rest
and go through another
set. A slight stretching or
burning sensation in
your buttocks and hips is
a sign that your muscles
are benefiting from the
exercise.

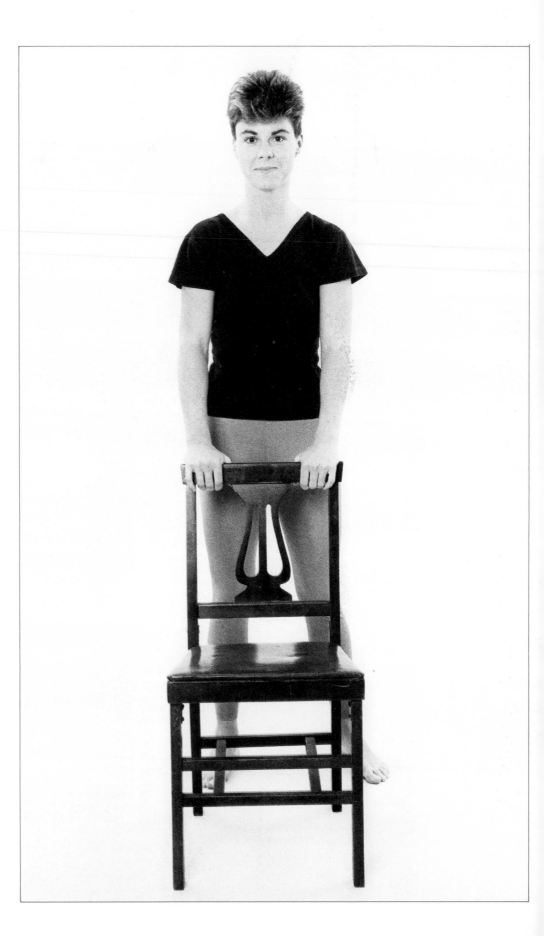

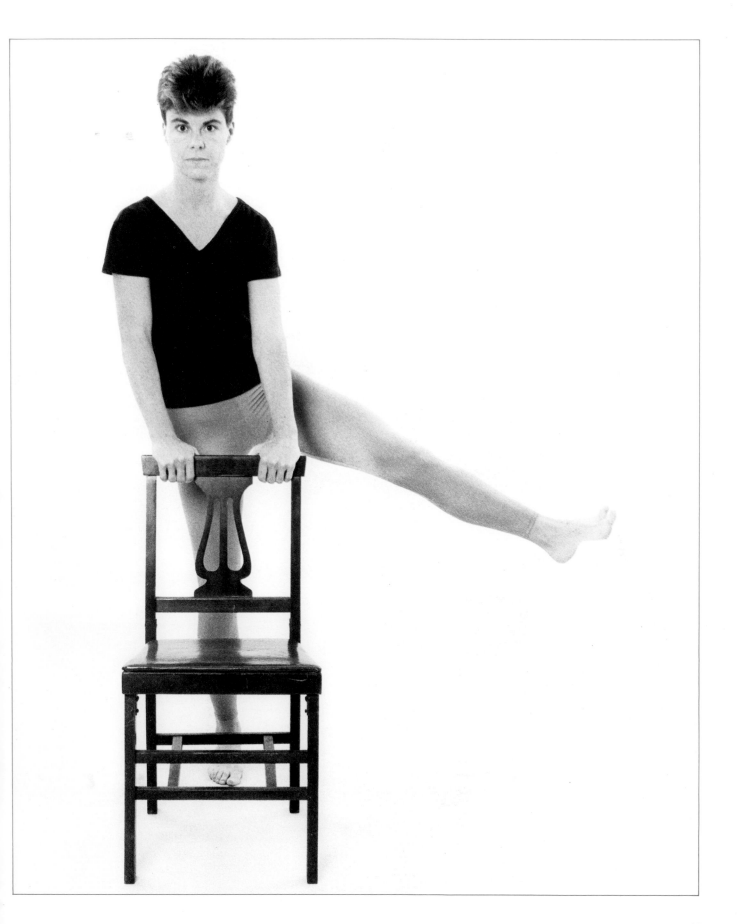

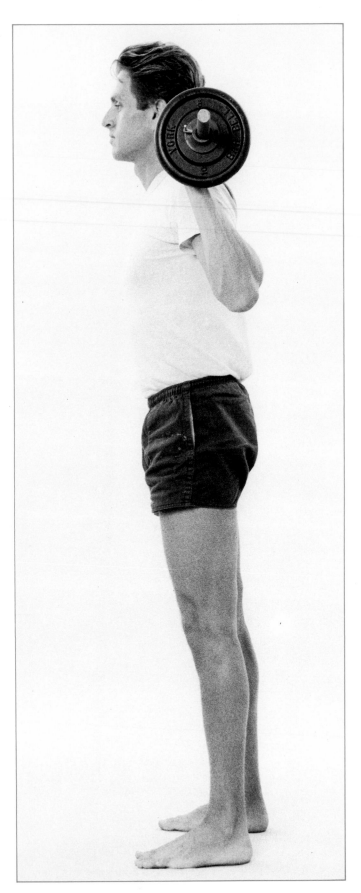

Calf Exercises

1. Barbell Lunge

(One set, 10 repetitions with each leg)
Place a barbell across your shoulders and behind your neck. Balance it in place by grasping the barbell bar in an overhand grip. If the weight hurts your neck, wrap the bar with a towel. Place your feet a few inches apart; hold your back straight. Now, keeping your right leg

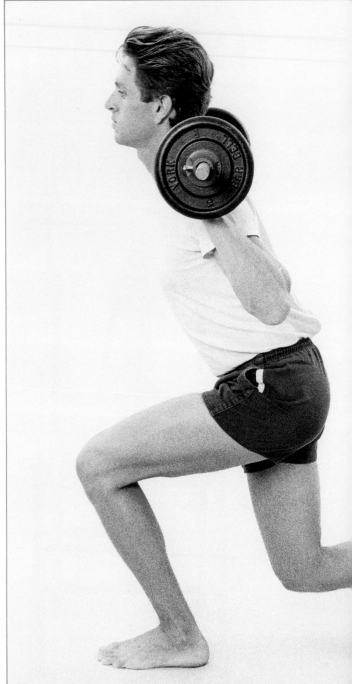

only slightly bent, step forward 2½ to 3 ft with your left foot. Then slowly bend your left leg as fully as possible while keeping your torso erect. At the bottom point of the movement

your right knee should be about 12 ins behind your left ankle. Push yourself back to the starting point and repeat the movement with your right foot forward. Alternate forward legs

for the required number of reps, counting one repetition each time both feet have been forward. Remember to go easy on the poundage you use for this exercise. Increase

poundage *only* after you have mastered this movement and feel minimal resistance from the barbell.

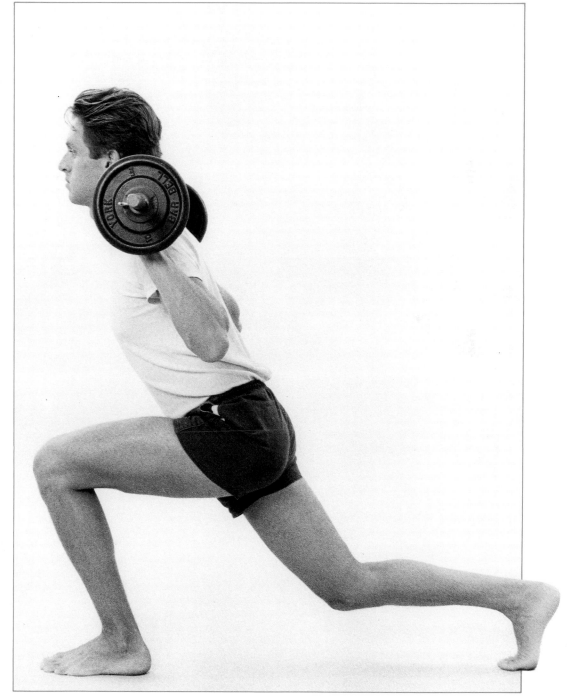

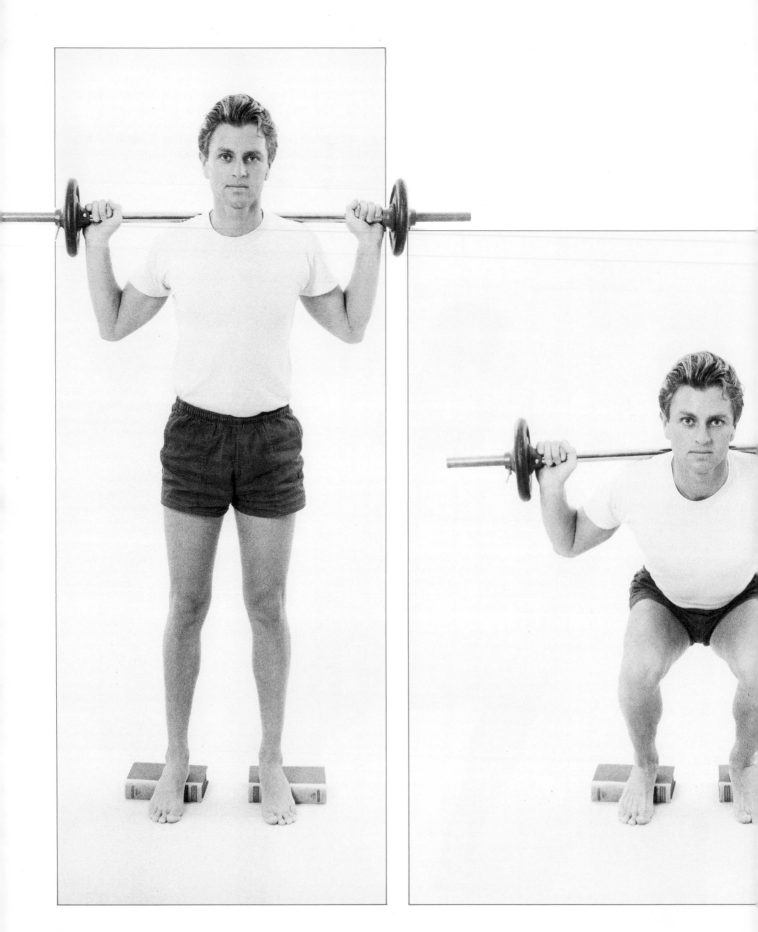

2. Barbell Squat

(One set, 15 repetitions) As with the Lunge, use light poundage at first for this exercise. The starting position for this is similar to that of the Lunge. Place the barbell across your shoulders and behind your neck. Balance it by holding the bar in an overhand grip. Place feet shoulder-width apart, toes pointed slightly outwards. Now, focusing on a point at shoulder height, with torso erect, slowly bend your knees and sink into a full squatting position. Without bouncing as you squat, slowly rise to starting position. If you have trouble keeping your balance during this exercise, stand with your heels on a 2 x 4 in block of wood — or a thick book — as you do the squats.

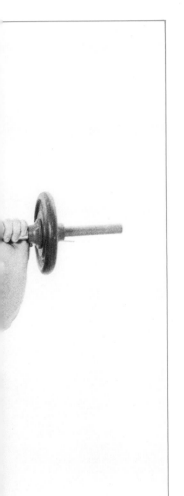

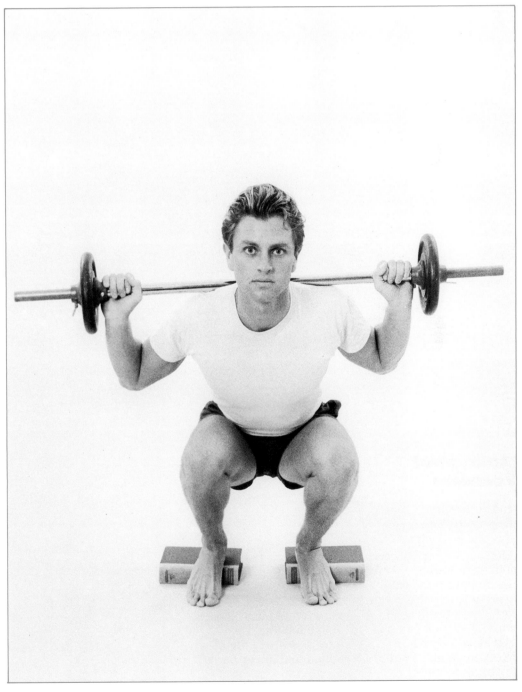

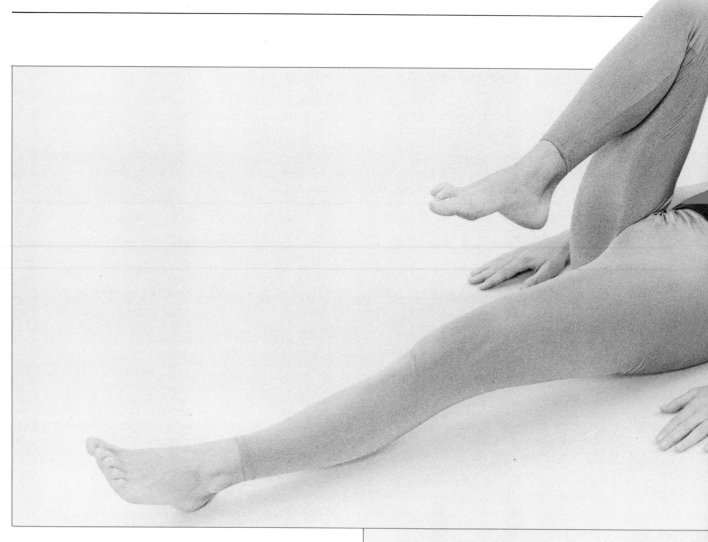

Abdominal Exercises

1. Alternating Leg Crunches

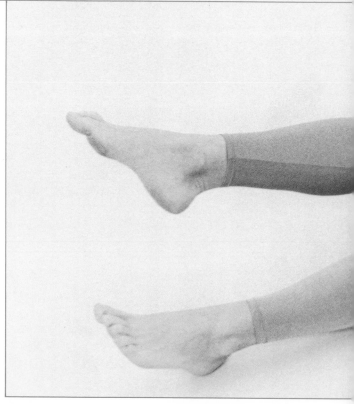

(One set, 20 repetitions with each leg)
Lie on your back with arms at sides. Bring your right knee as close to your chest as it can go, and slowly extend it back out again. Your lower abdominal muscles will feel a pull as you do this. Drop your leg to the floor for one repetition. Switch to your left leg; do 20 reps with each leg. This exercise also promotes spinal and lower back flexibility.

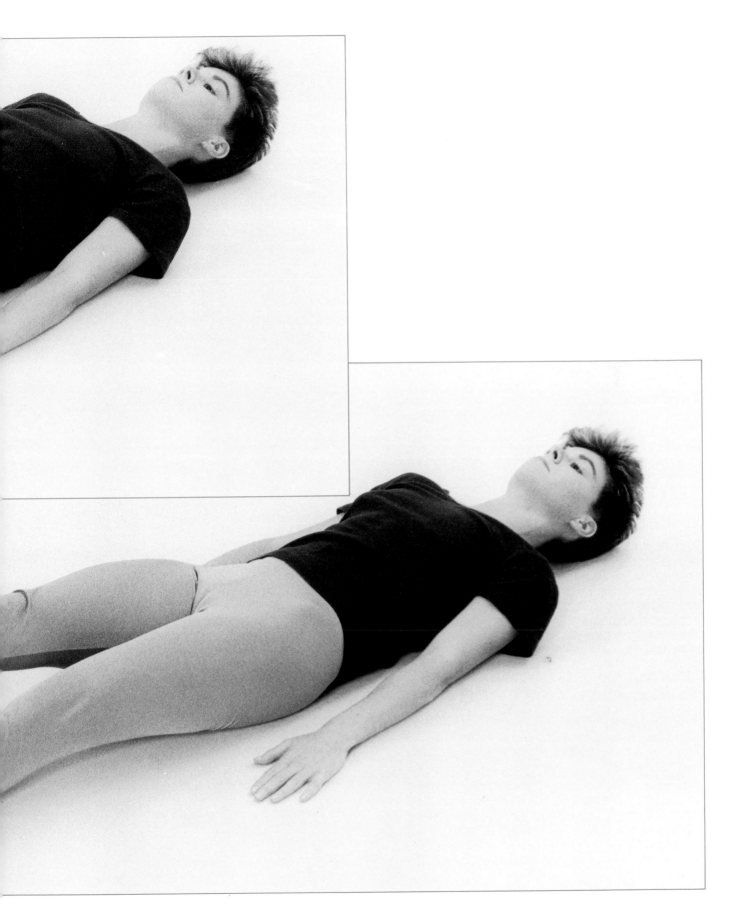

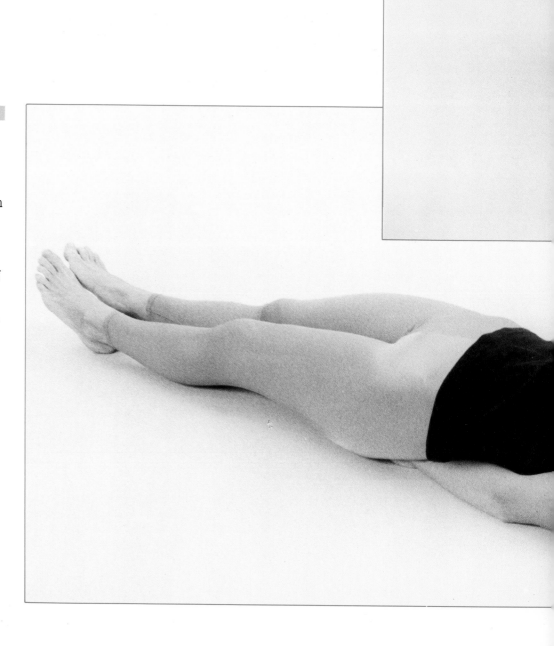

2. Leg Raises

(One set, 15 repetitions)
Lie on your back with
your hands tucked
underneath your
buttocks, palms down on
the floor. Keep your
legs and feet together.
Now, lift your legs 6 ins
off the floor and hold
them there for a count of
three seconds. Steadily
lower them to the floor
for one repetition. Try to
increase the number of
repetitions you can do
each time.

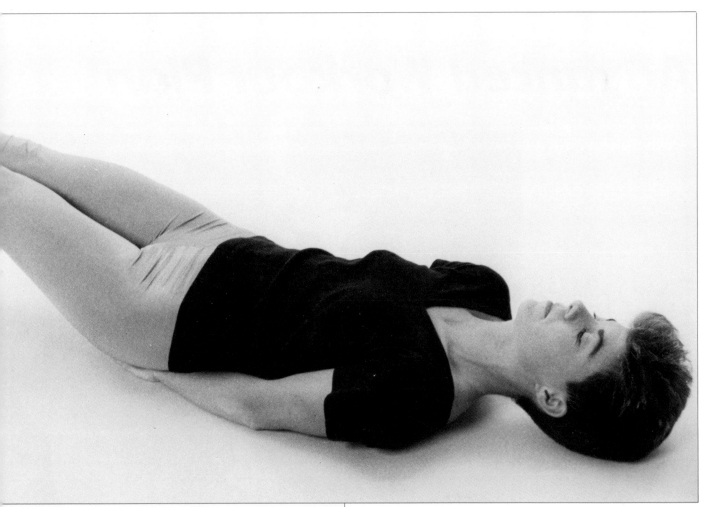

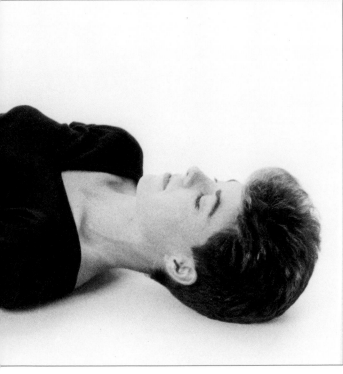

Chapter 5

Advanced Workout Plan

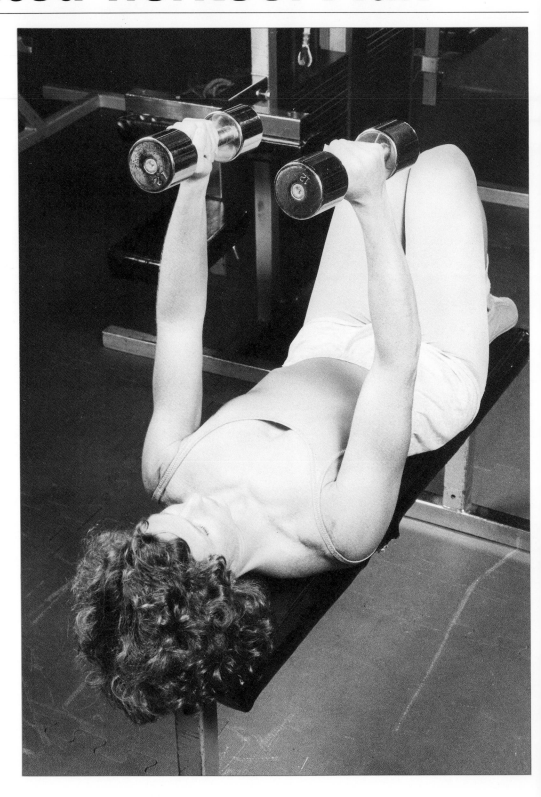

Chest Exercises.

1. Dumb-bell Flies

(One set, 20 repetitions) Lie on your back on a bench, your feet spread wide. Hold the two dumb-bells up over your chest, with arms bent slightly at the elbows. Keeping your arms bent, lower the weights to the level of the bench (your elbows should drop beneath it) and bring them smoothly back up, keeping tension in your chest muscles. The dumb-bells should be slightly apart at the top of the repetition.

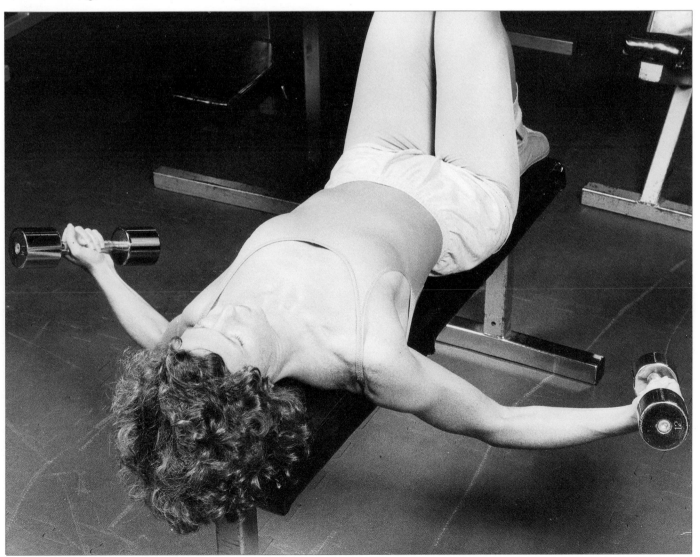

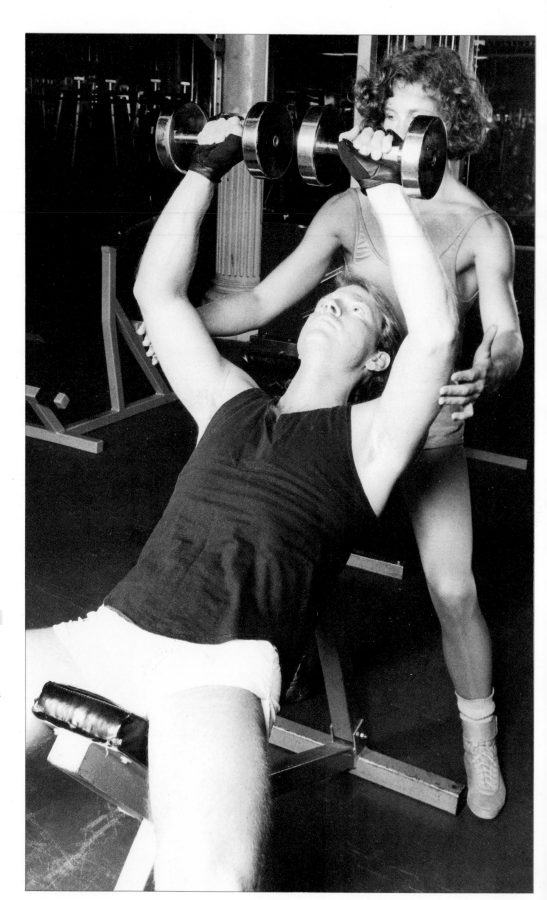

2. Dumb-bell Press

(One set, 20 repetitions)
Sit in an inclining chair,
your feet spread wide.
Hold the two dumb-bells
overhead. Inhale and
lower slowly so the
dumb-bells are above
your shoulders; your
arms forming L-shapes
(your elbows should be
at shoulder-level). Now
exhale as you raise the
dumb-bells up using
your chest muscles. To
do this exercise
properly at first you
may need a spotter.

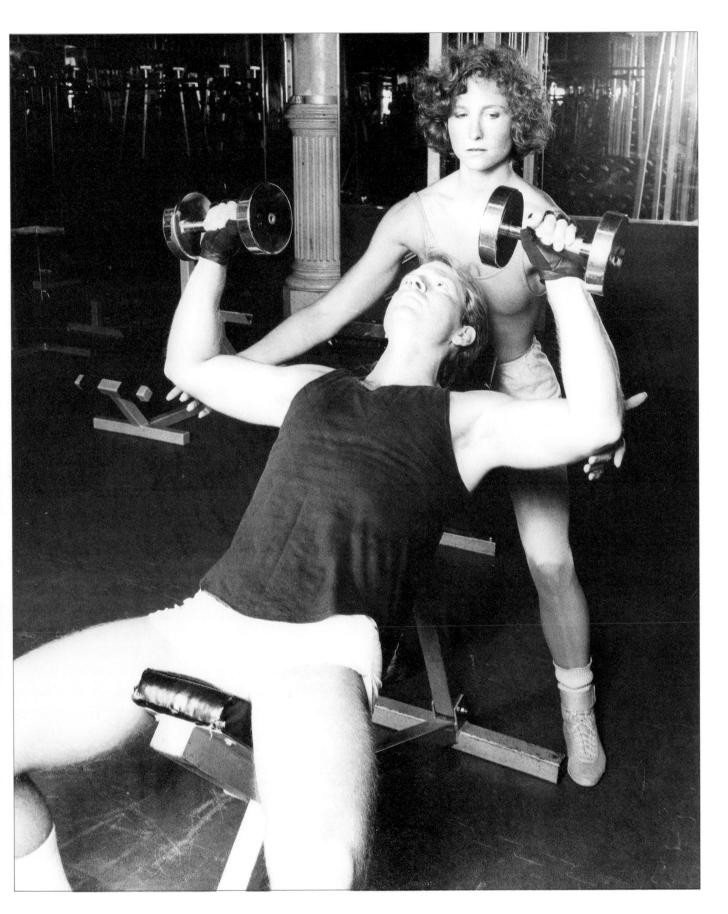

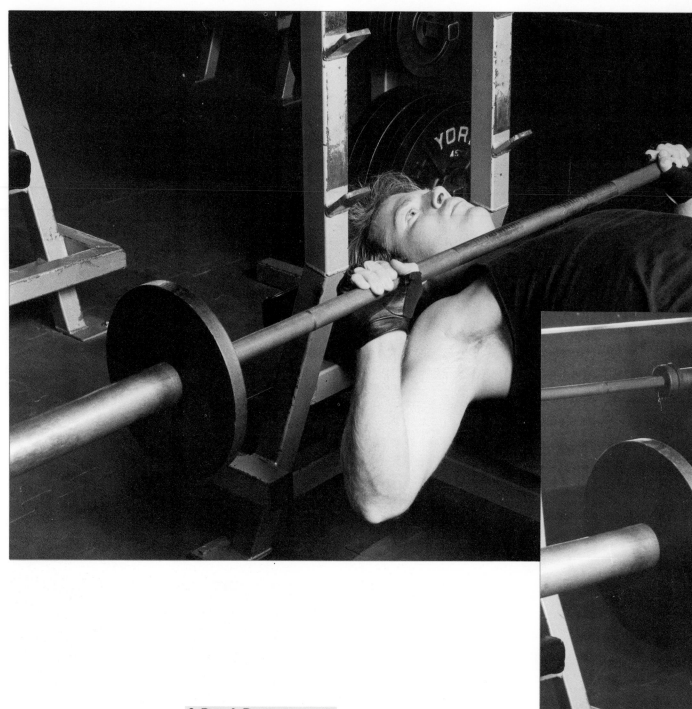

3. Bench Press

(One set, 20 repetitions) Lie on your back on the bench, feet spread wide, holding the bar on your chest in as wide a grip as you can make between the weights. Raise the bar an inch or two off your chest and use that position as the bottom of each repetition in order to keep tension on the pectoral muscles. Inhale as you lower the weight; exhale as you raise it to the top point of the rep.

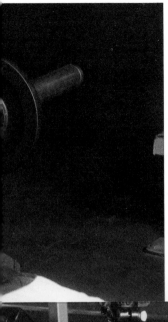

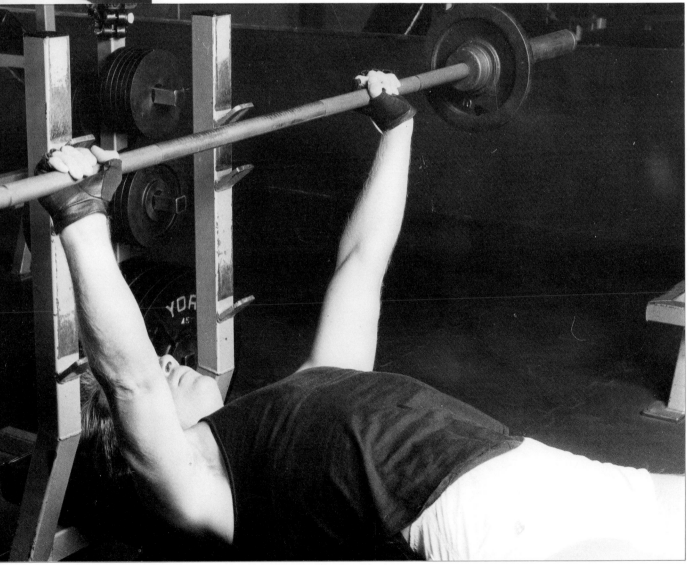

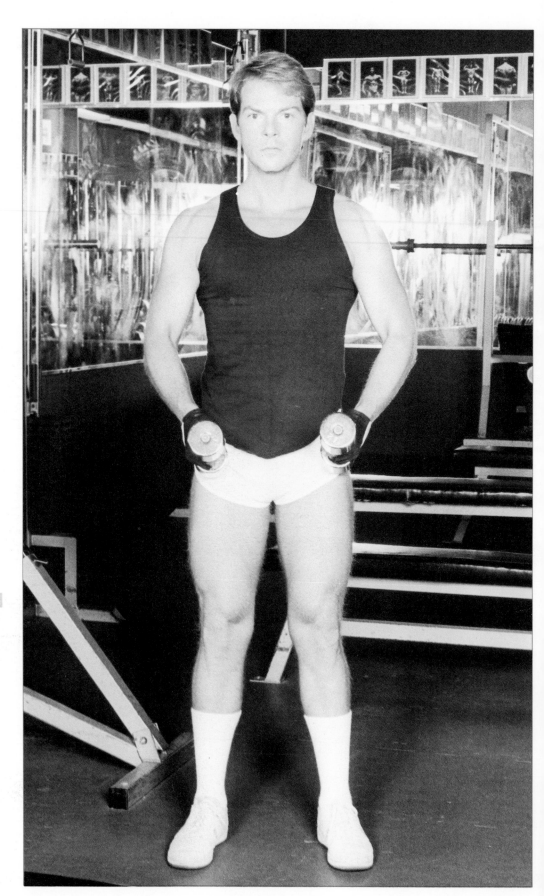

Shoulder Exercises

1. Side Laterals

(One set, 20 repetitions) Stand with your feet shoulder-width apart. Hold the two dumb-bells in front of your hips, palms facing each other, with arms bent a little at the elbows and leaning slightly forward at the waist. Now raise dumb-bells up to shoulder level; steadily lower them to original position. Remember to inhale on the relaxation phase of the movement, and to exhale on the resistance phase.

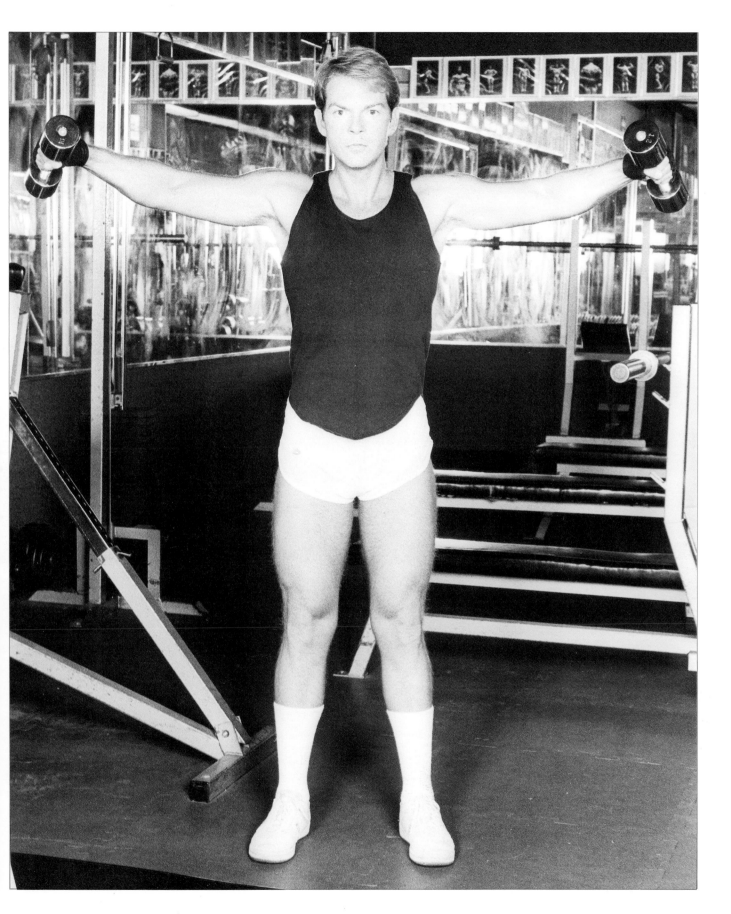

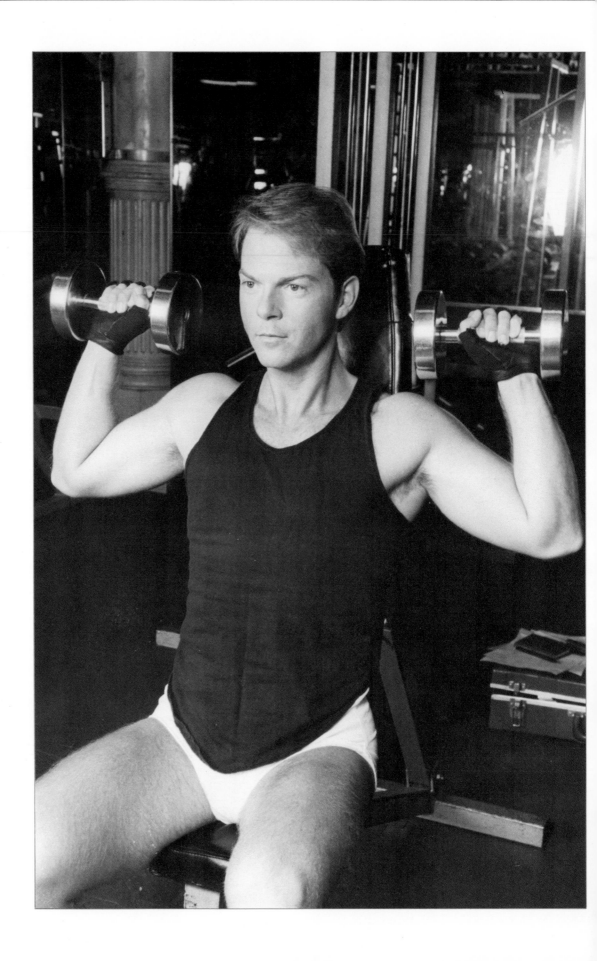

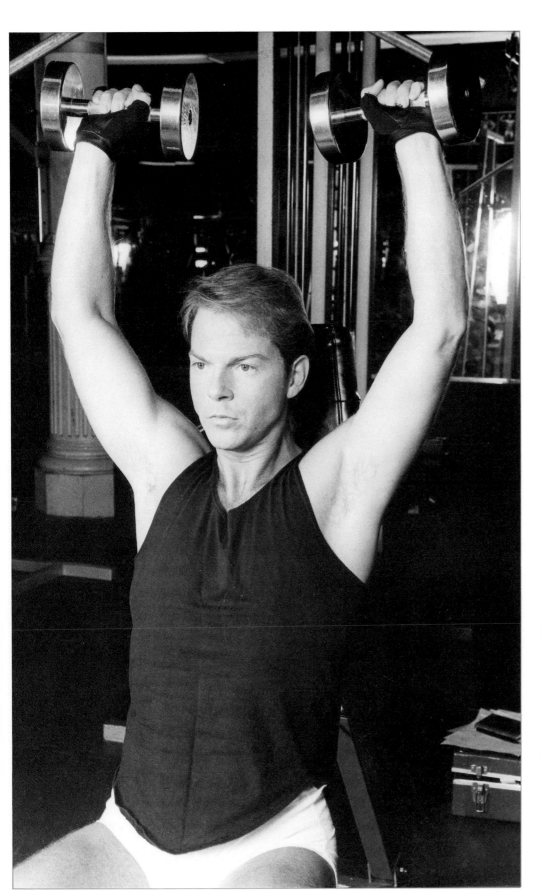

2. Seated Dumb-bell Press

(One set, 20 repetitions) Sit in a straight-backed chair holding the two dumb-bells above your shoulders as pictured. Exhale as you slowly raise the dumb-bell overhead, feeling the tension in the top of your shoulders. Bring the dumb-bells within a few inches of each other, then lower slowly to original position, inhaling as you go.

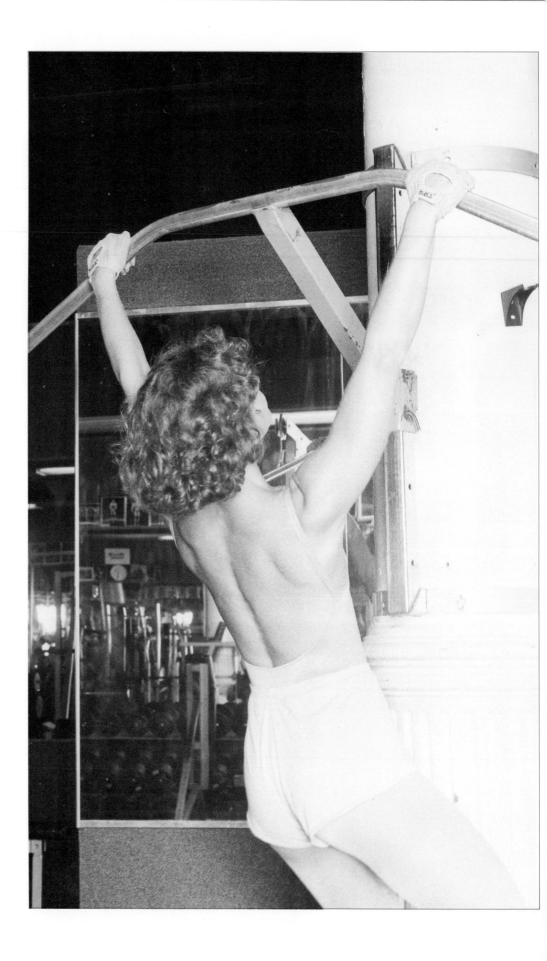

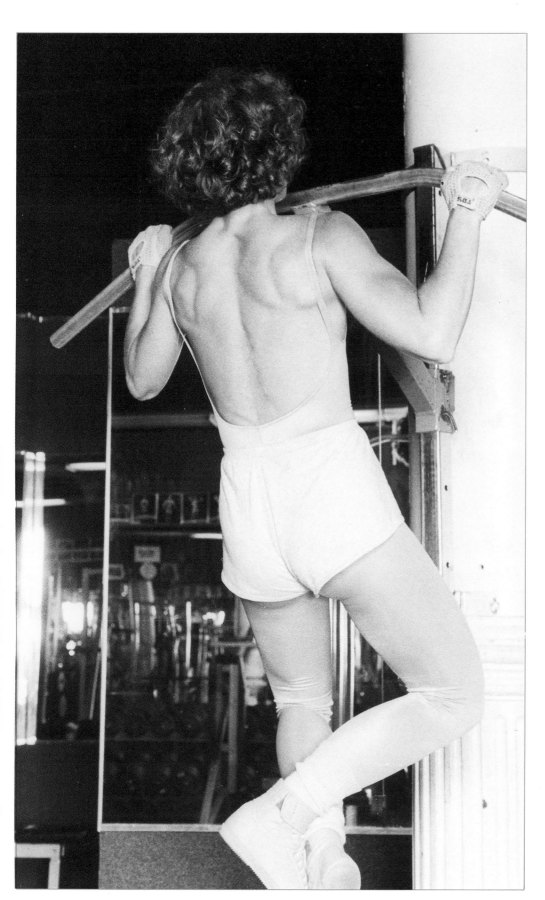

Back Exercises

1. Chins

(One set, 10 repetitions) Take hold of the chinning bar in an overhand grip as pictured, your hands about 3 ft apart. Lift your feet off the ground and cross your legs behind you at the ankles. Pull yourself straight up, exhaling as you rise, until your chin hovers above the bar. Lower yourself slowly for one repetition.

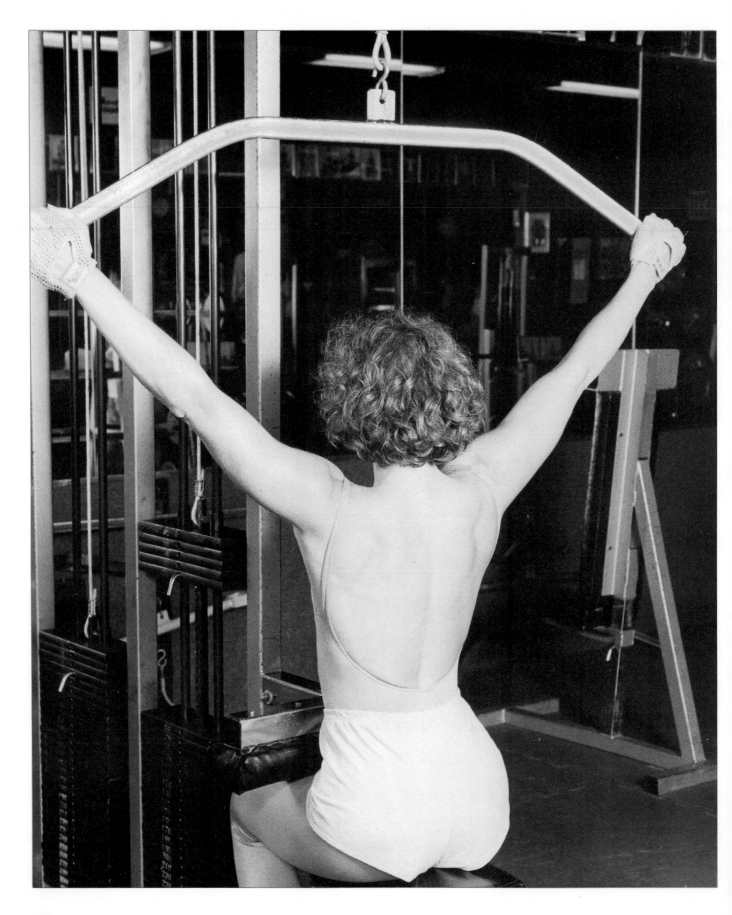

2. Lat Pull-downs

(One set, 15 repetitions) Sitting up straight with your body beneath the bar, grasp the bar's grips so that your arms are extended. Keeping your head erect, pull the bar smoothly down behind your neck, touching the backs of your shoulders, and let it smoothly back up. Maintaining proper breathing form as you go will give your muscles the extra push they need to lower the bar.

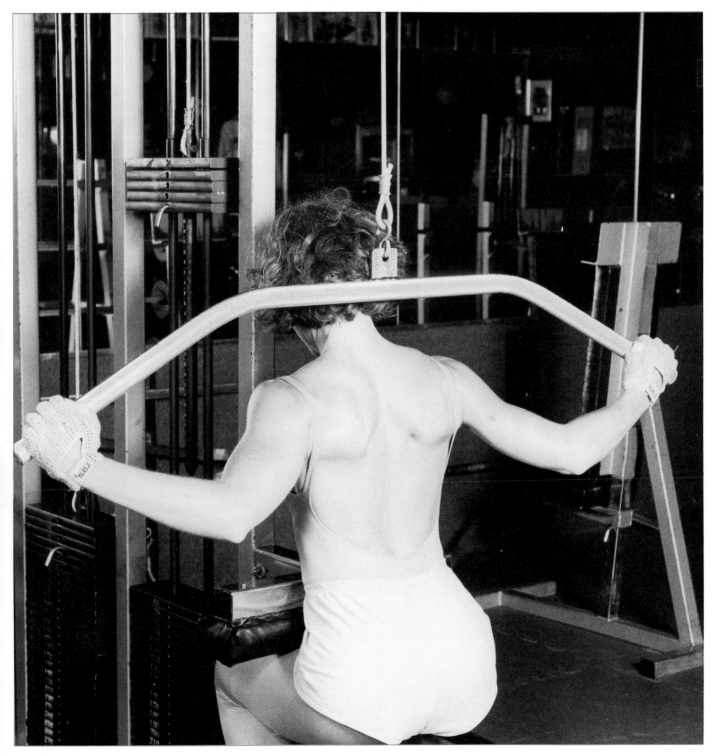

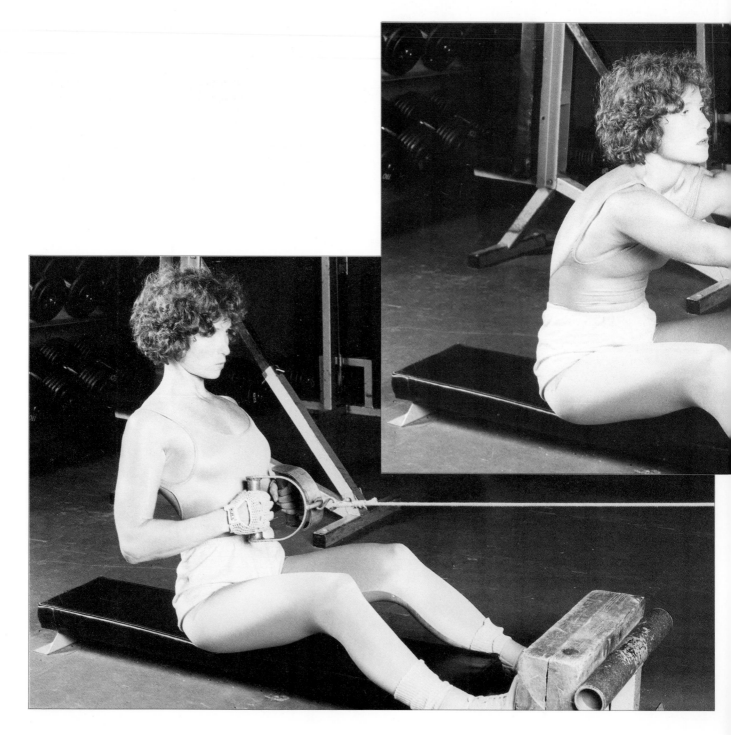

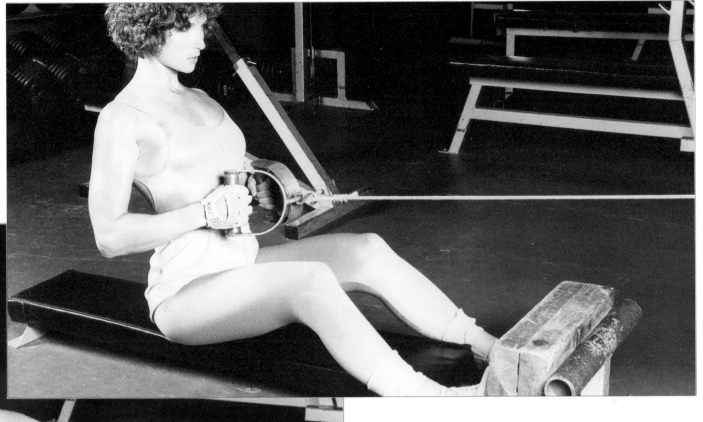

3. Low Cable Rows

(One set, 15 repetitions) Sit up straight on the machine's bench, with your legs bent at the knees and your feet braced. Grasp the cables against your stomach and slowly extend your arms to release the weight, bending your upper body forward as you go. When the weight is nearly touching the bottom of the machine steadily pull the cables back towards your stomach and sit up straight into original position.

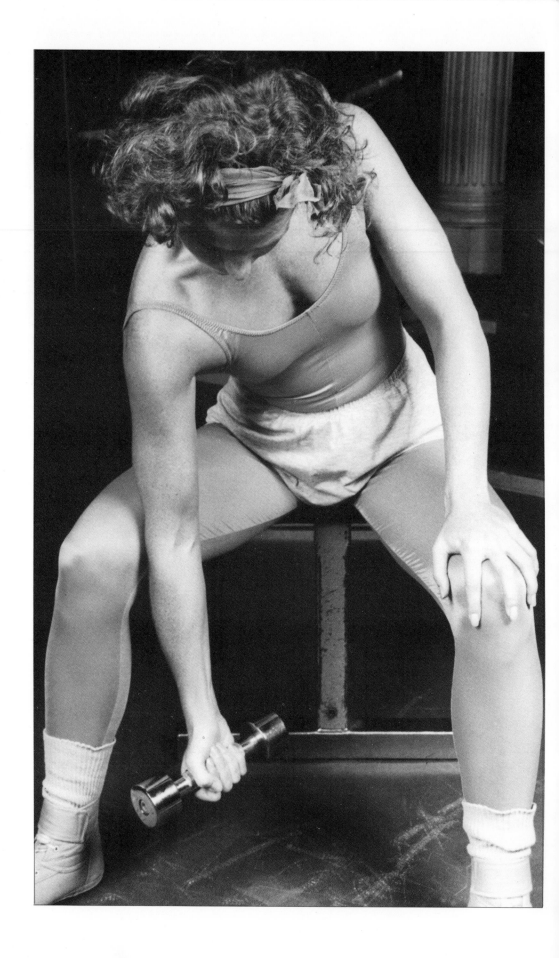

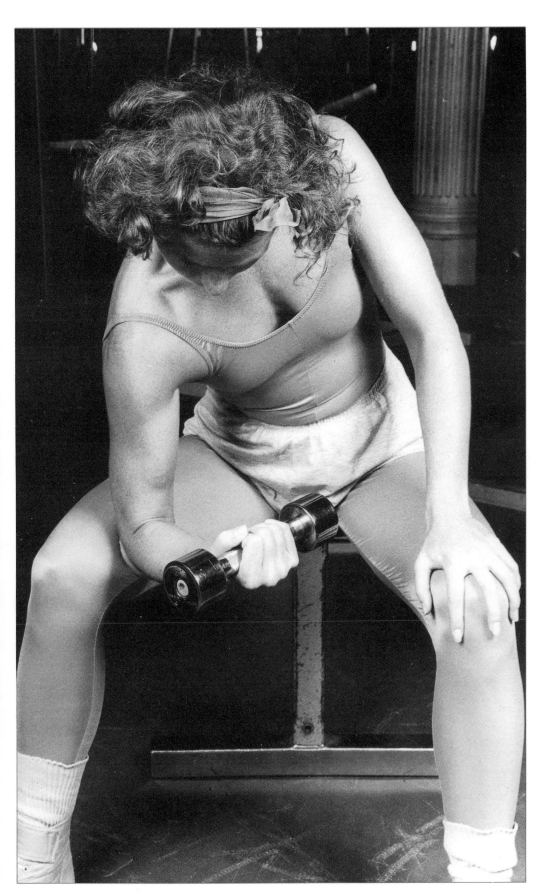

Biceps Exercises

1. Biceps Concentration Curl

(One set, 10 repetitions with each arm)
This exercise accentuates the peak of your biceps. Sit at the end of a flat exercise bench with feet about 6 ins wider on each side than shoulder-width. Grasp a dumb-bell in your right hand. Lean forward, pinning your right elbow against the inside of your right leg near your knee. Turn your wrist so that your palm is facing directly away from your leg and keep it in this position throughout the movement. Hold your left hand on your left knee. From this position, slowly curl the dumb-bell up to your shoulder so that your biceps peak. Lower it back to original position and repeat the movement. (On all exercises for one arm or one leg be sure to do an equal number of repetitions and sets for each limb.) Do 10 repetitions with this arm, then switch to your left arm for 10 more.

2. Double Arm Biceps Curl

(One set, 20 repetitions) Sit in an inclining chair that is at a 35° angle holding two dumb-bells at your sides, slightly below hip level, in an underhand grip. Now, slowly raise the dumb-bells up to a point in front of your shoulders, keeping your arms close to your sides as you go. Lower the dumb-bells steadily to complete the repetition.

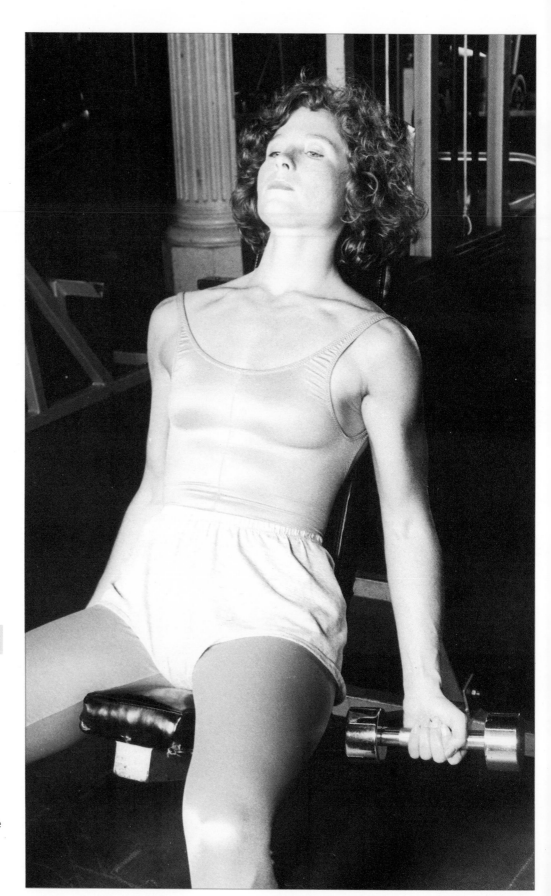

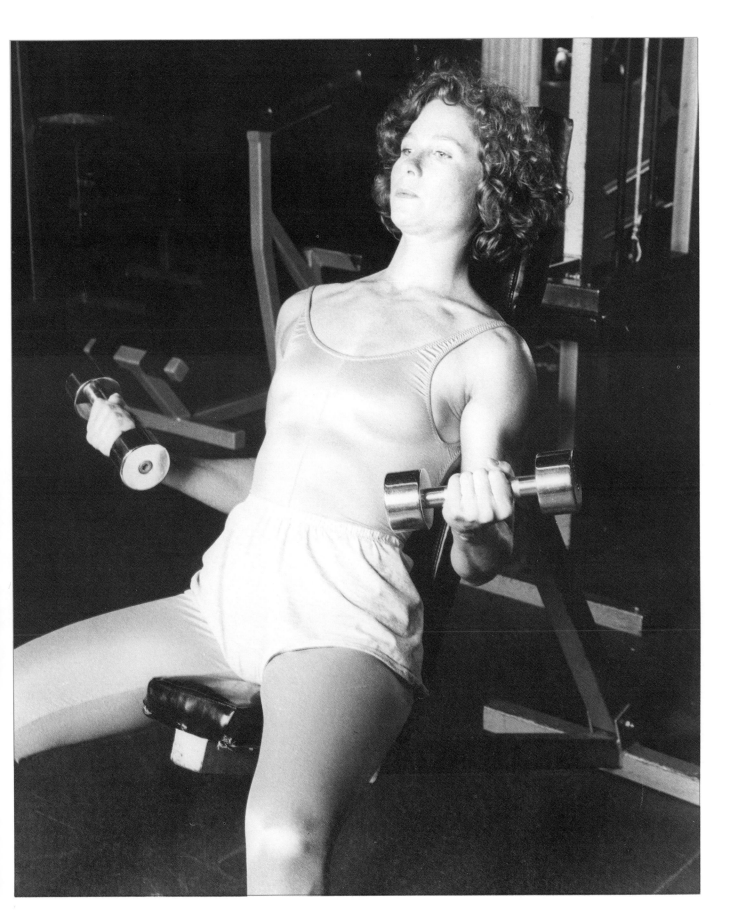

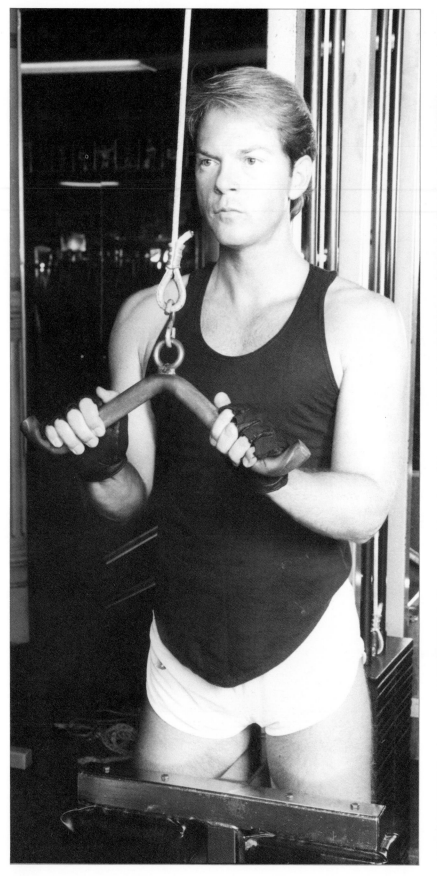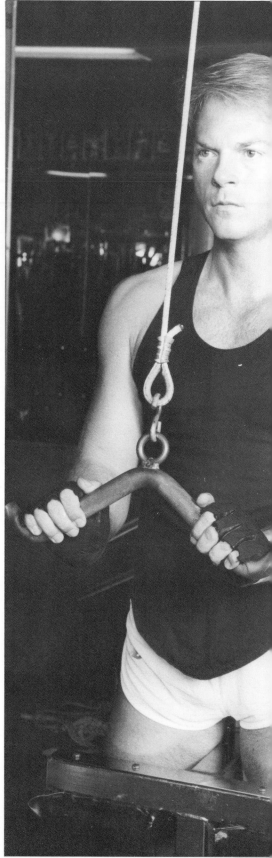

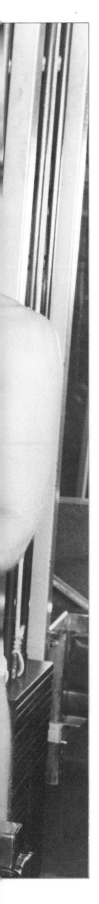

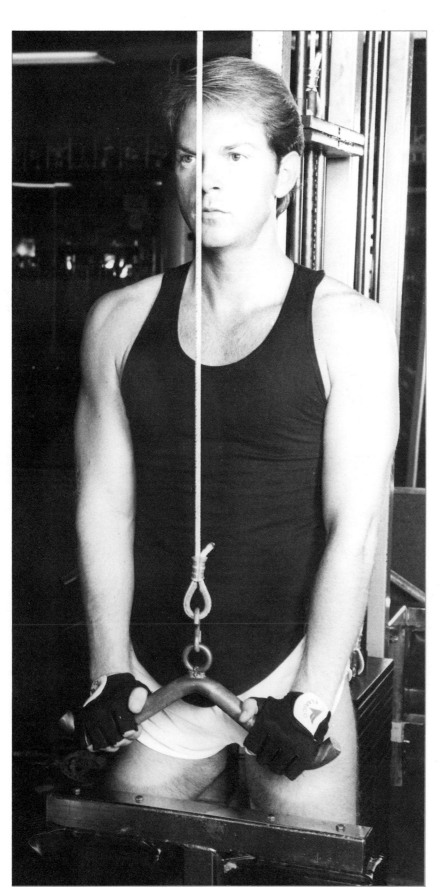

Triceps Exercises

1. Triceps Pull-downs

(One set, 20 repetitions) Stand with your feet about shoulder-width apart and grip the bar as pictured. Keeping your back and upper arm straight, and your elbows close to your sides and still, push the bar down towards the floor to just above your waist. (This is the top position for each repetition.) Now continue to push the bar down, feeling the strain in your triceps, until your elbows are nearly locked. Then slowly let it up again to just above your waist to complete the repetition.

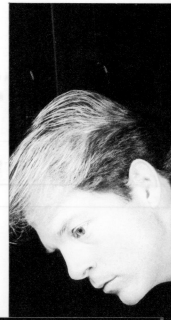

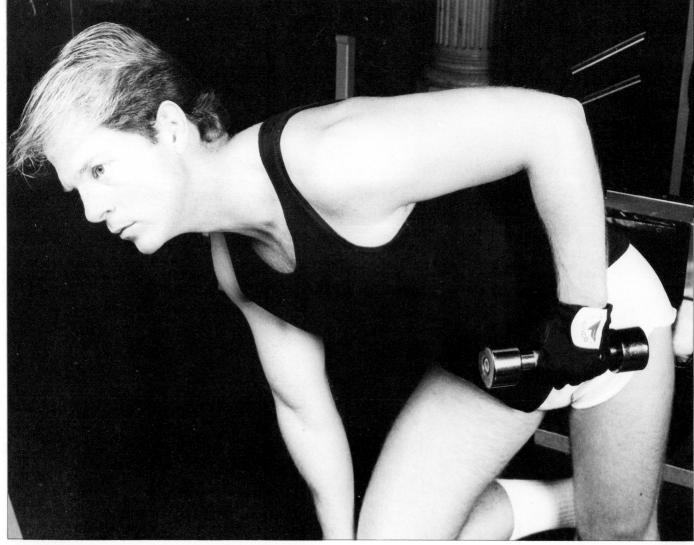

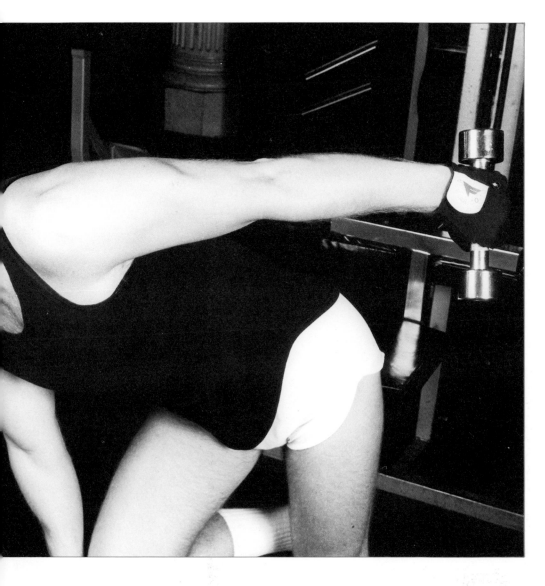

2. Triceps Dumb-bell Kickback

(One set, 20 repetitions with each arm)
Brace your right arm and knee as pictured on the end of an exercise bench. Hold a dumb-bell in your left hand at hip height; your upper arm should be slanted straight back. Now, using only the muscles in the back of your upper arm, slowly extend the weight backwards until your elbow has locked. Steadily bring it back in for one repetition.

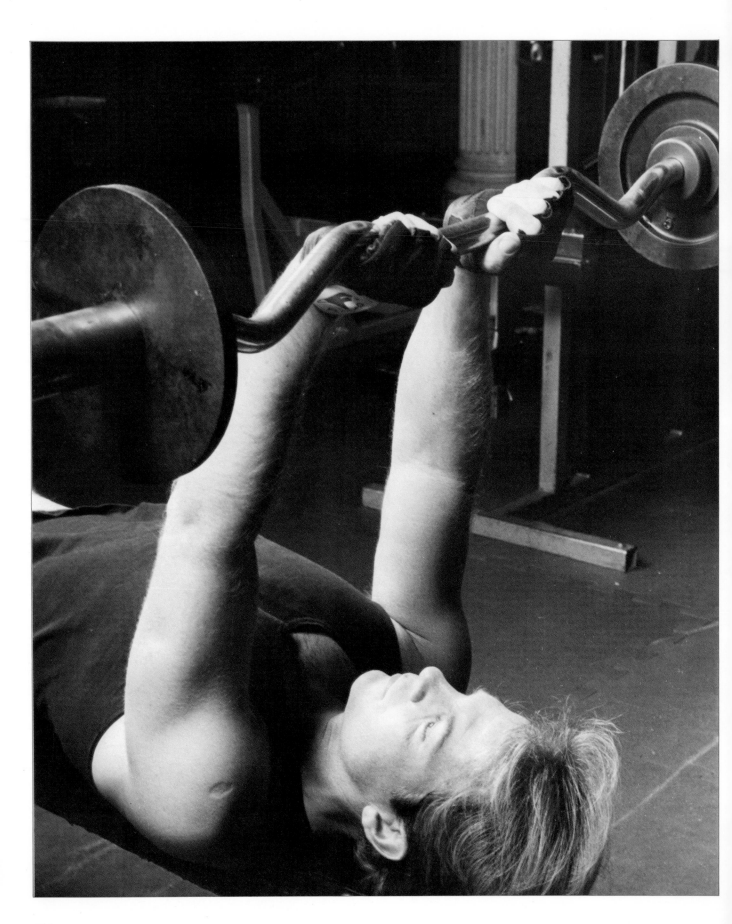

3. Overhead E-Z Curls

(One set, 20 repetitions) Lie on your back on an exercise bench. Take a narrow overgrip in the middle of an E-Z curl bar (leave about 6 ins of space between your index fingers). Now extend your arms directly above your shoulder joints, exhaling as you push up. Keeping your upper arms motionless, slowly bend your arms and lower the bar downwards so that it almost touches your forehead. Use your triceps' power to return the bar to the starting position above your head.

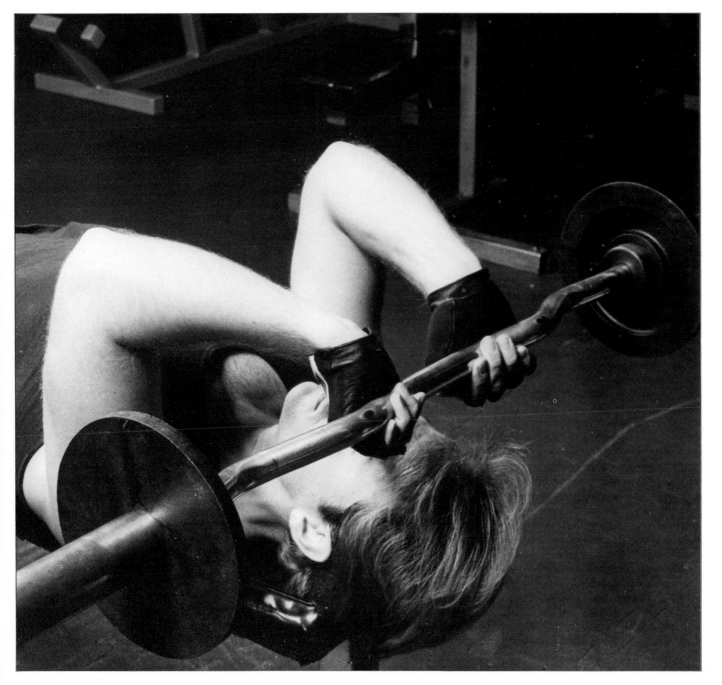

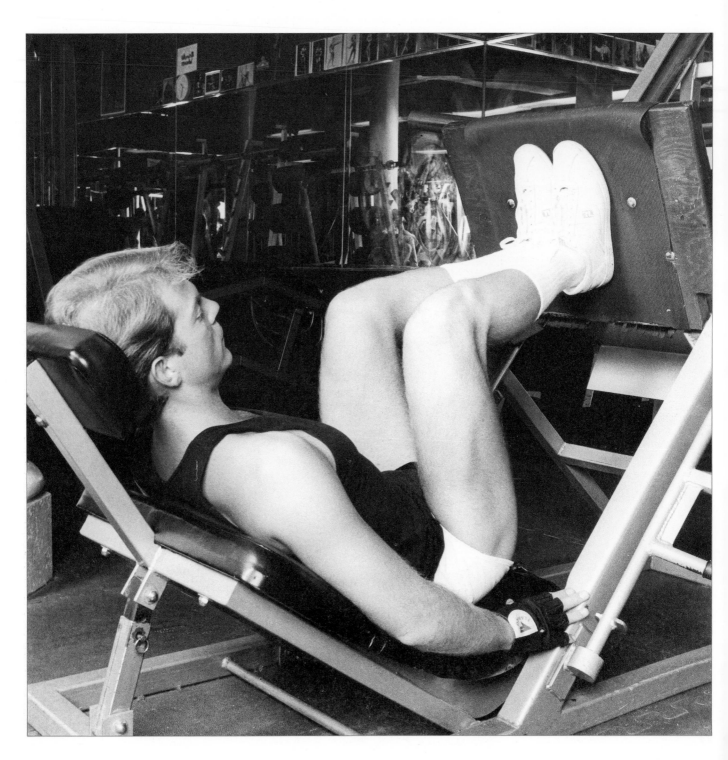

Leg Exercises

1. Leg Press

(One set, 20 repetitions) Sitting in a leg machine chair, with straight back and hands on grips, place your feet together on the weight with knees bent — your knees should be a few inches from your chest. Now, slowly extend your legs, exhaling as you go, until the weight has been pushed so far that your knees are nearly locked. Smoothly return to original position for one repetition.

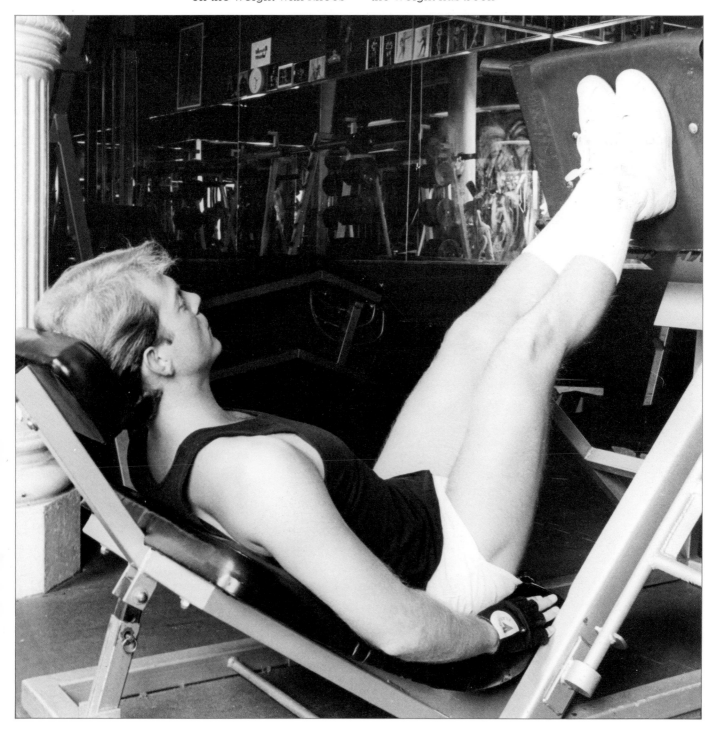

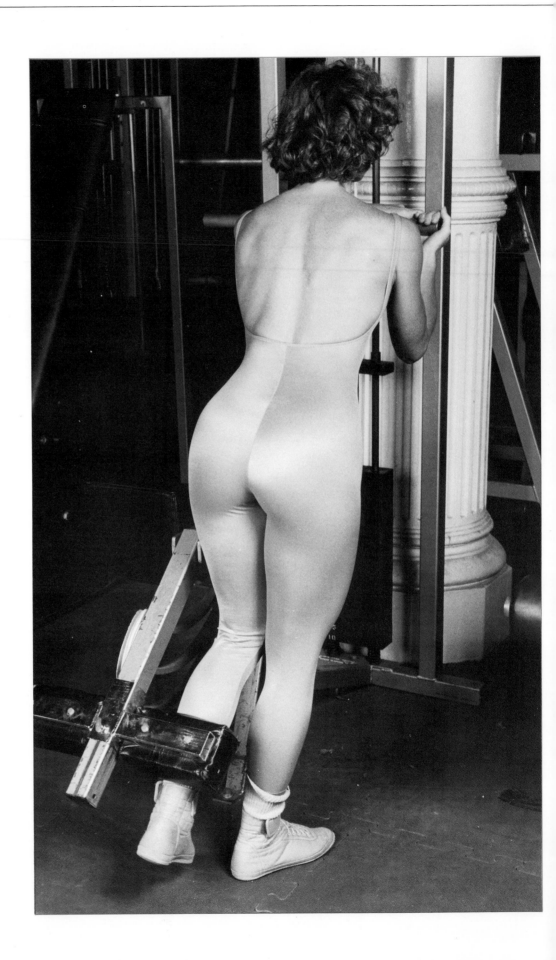

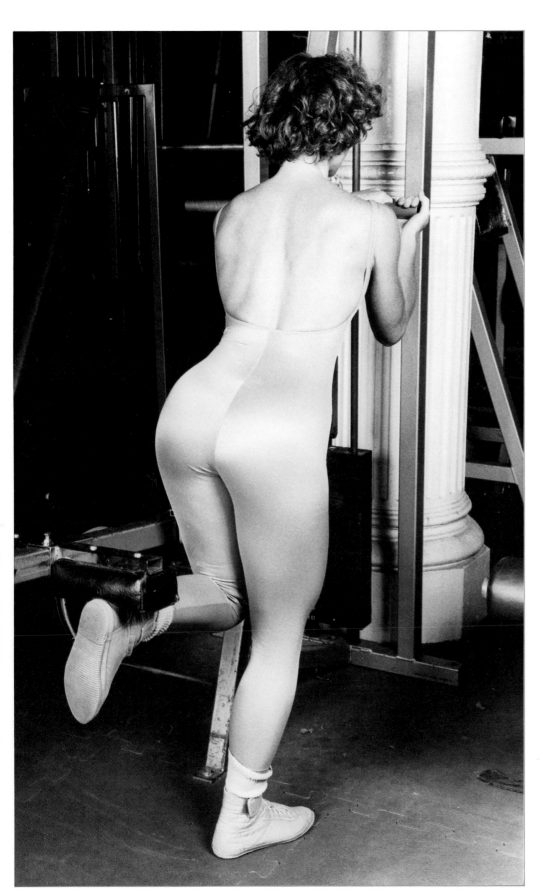

2. Standing Leg Curl

(One set, 20 repetitions with each leg)
This exercise tones the back biceps muscle in your thigh. Stand in front of the leg machine, bent slightly forward at the waist, grasping the bar in an underhand grip. Brace your left leg in front of the weight so that your calf lies against it. Now slowly push back the weight as far as you can, exhaling and feeling the pull as you go. Lower steadily to complete the repetition. Do 20 repetitions with this leg and switch to the other for 20 more.

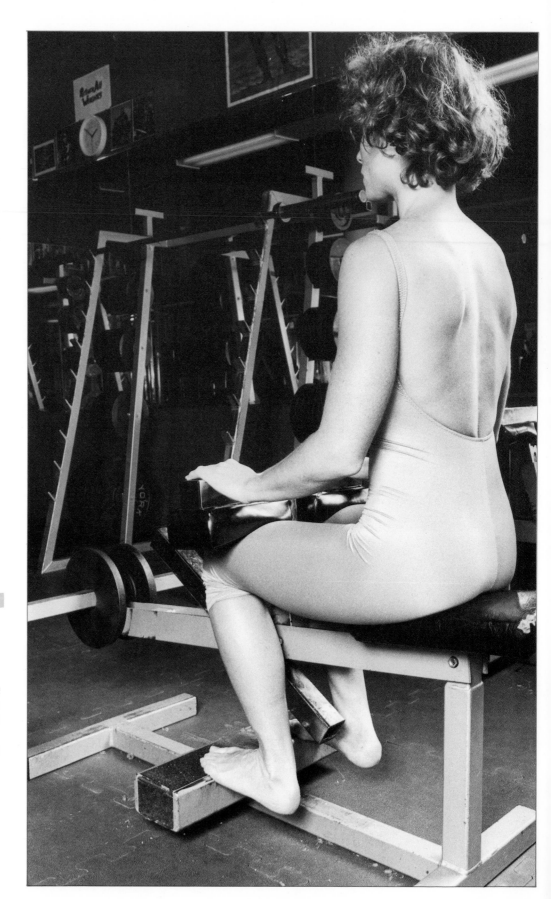

Calf Exercises

1. Seated Calf Raise

(One set, 20 repetitions)
Sitting up straight in the
calf machine's seat,
place feet a few inches
apart as shown, with toes
and the balls of your fee
firmly on the metal plate
Pull the padded bar of
the machine over the top
of your knees. Rise up
on your toes far enough
to push the weight and
release it. Now drop
your heels as far below
toe level as possible,
and slowly push up and
drop down as far as you
can go on your toes.

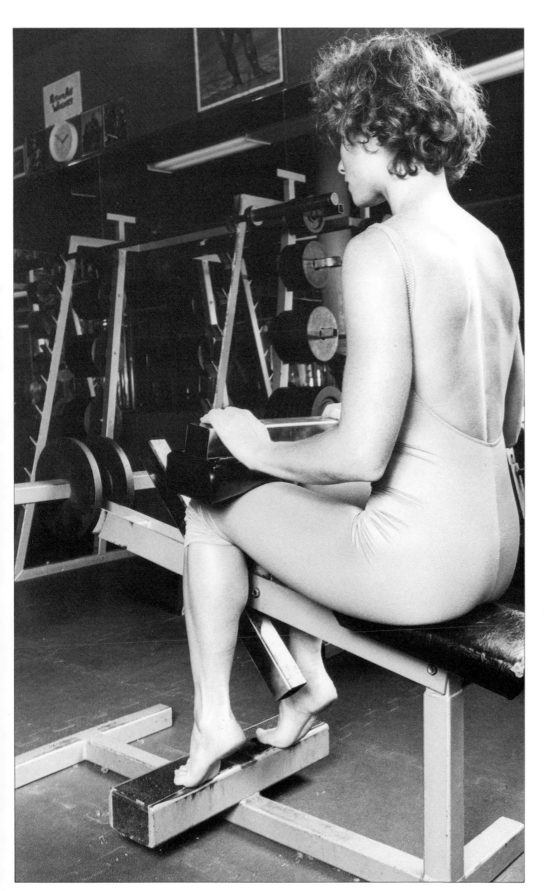

2. Barbell Lunge
(Not illustrated)

(One set, 10 repetitions with each leg)
This is a variation on Intermediate Calf Exercise 1. Follow the method detailed there, only use increased poundage to make the exercise more challenging.

3. Barbell Squat
(Not illustrated)

(One set, 15 repetitions)
A variation on Intermediate Calf Exercise 2. The Barbell Squat can build more muscle if you add 10 lbs or more to the bar. If you are especially interested in building more muscle and strength in your calves, try doing two or more sets of barbell squats with a brief (two minute) rest interval in between sets.

Abdominal Exercises

1. Abdominal Crunches

(One set, 25 repetitions) Lie on your back with hands clasped behind your head, legs over a flat exercise bench, thighs perpendicular to the floor. This exercise is performed not unlike a sit-up, except the form is more exacting. As you do the movement, you must concentrate on simultaneously doing these four things:
— use lower abdominal muscles to raise your hips from the floor.
— tense the upper abdominals to raise your shoulders up off the floor.
— try to force your shoulders towards your pelvis, thereby 'crunching' or shortening your torso.
— exhale forcefully as you raise yourself off the floor.

If you perform the exercise correctly, you will feel a strong contraction in your frontal abdominals. Slowly lower yourself back to the floor for one rep.

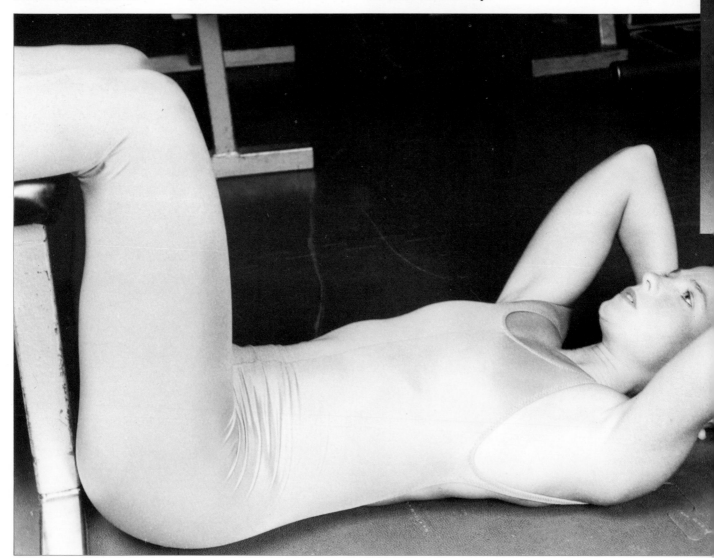

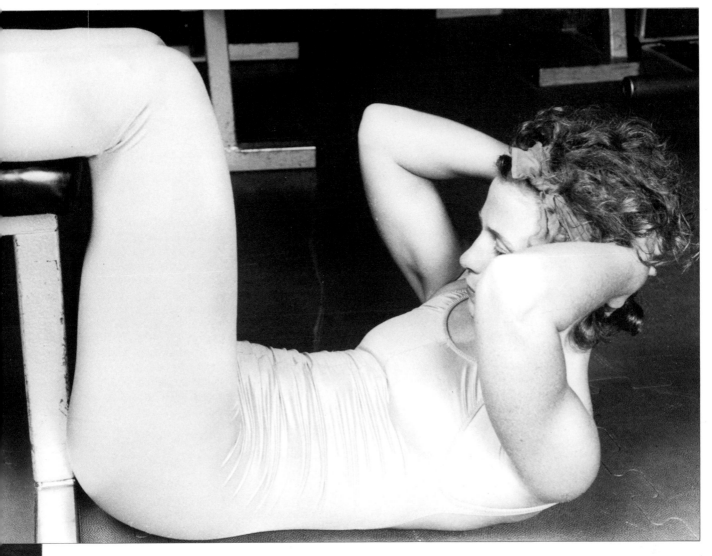

2. Leg Raises
(Not illustrated)

(Two sets, 15 repetitions each)
Follow the instructions for Intermediate Abdominal Exercise 2. Take a rest interval of three minutes in between sets.

Chapter 6

Keeping your shape

Training Tips

It's wise to set a fixed workout schedule for yourself so that your body has enough time to rest and re-charge itself in between weight training sessions. Some people prefer exercising before they go to work, as it energizes them for the day ahead. Others like to wait until the evening to use their workout as a physical and mental release. One drawback to training in the morning is that in the beginning you may feel very fatigued after working out. Once your body adjusts to the new demands of your exercise regime, however, you'll feel revitalized afterwards no matter what time of day you work out. The key at the beginning is *patience*: it will take weeks for your body to recondition itself, but your reward will be a better body and improved strength, endurance and flexibility.

The Beginning and Intermediate programs in this book can be done anywhere in your home, office, hotel room, etc. All you really need is a few feet of open space. Doing the exercises in front of a mirror is especially helpful, as you can keep an eye on your form as you work out, ensuring that you perform the movements properly. Your exercise area should also be well ventilated — you'll be breathing hard and working up a sweat — so circulating air is an absolute must.

Clothing and Accessories Guidelines

'What to wear for exercise is primarily a matter of personal preference,' says Nancy Pollak, a New York clothing designer specializing in high fashion athletic bodywear. Nancy, herself a dedicated bodybuilder, tests her designs by working out in them and then altering the cut and fabric as needed. She suggests you consider the following before suiting up:
• Your clothing must allow a free range of movement for your body parts. Any constricting garments are to be avoided. It's alright to wear tight-fitting clothes, but the fabric must be able to stretch with your movements.
• Select clothes that are made of absorbent fabrics, especially if you tend to perspire profusely. Cotton shirts, shorts and sweatpants are recommended. You

might also want to wear cotton wristbands and a headband to absorb excess perspiration.
• Wear clothes in colours that make you feel good — your favourite colours can be a psychological boost as you work out, and if you train in a gym, other people will appreciate your contribution to the atmosphere!
• Weightlifting gloves are useful aids for barbell and dumb-bell exercises. These fingerless mesh gloves are usually made of leather; they give you a better grip on your equipment and are a must for those who have sweaty palms or sensitive skin that callouses easily.
• Wear absorbent cotton socks and some kind of athletic shoe to protect your feet and ankles. Although Nancy likes to work out in white leather moccasins, most people who train with weights wear running shoes, tennis shoes, or high topped basketball sneakers for support.

Staying in Shape

One helpful strategy for keeping yourself in shape involves recording the specifics of each workout. Enter the exercise, the number of repetitions and sets done, and the poundage lifted. This way you can note your progress and pinpoint areas where you need to do more work. Charting your efforts in this way will also make it easier to set realistic goals for yourself. Many people who are on a combination weight training/weight loss program find that keeping track of everything they eat helps reinforce their willpower at meal times, so you may want to consider keeping a 'food journal' in addition to your workout notes. If restructuring your behaviour like this seems a little drastic, remember that the only way you can change yourself for the better is by establishing newer, more sensible living habits.

It's a widely acknowledged fact that you must train frequently in order to maintain, or improve, muscular strength and overall fitness. Most amateur bodybuilders recommend working out five times a week: two days in a row, then skip a day, then three days in a row, take a day off, and back to two days in a row. 'Working out fewer than three days a week, especially if you're a beginner, should be avoided at all costs,' says Beth Rubino, a competitive bodybuilder who has been training for only three years. 'Changing the shape of your body requires a consistent training

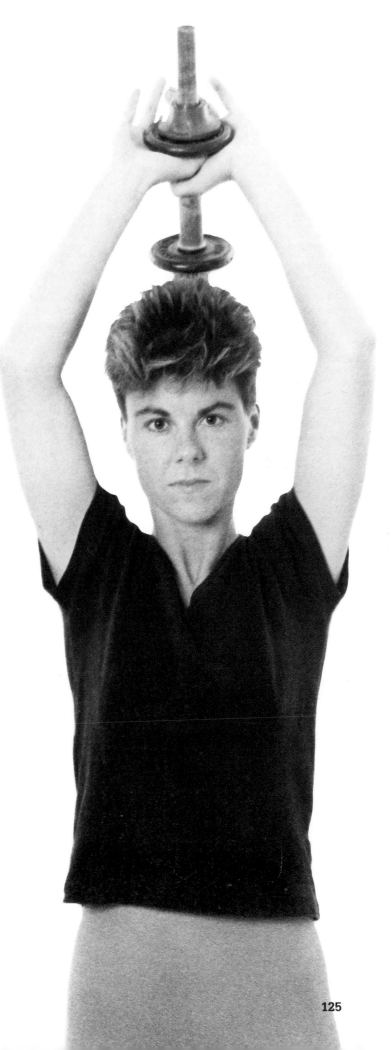

schedule. Committing yourself to working out five days a week will give you maximum results, which will in turn motivate you to continue and further improve your strength and appearance.'

On the other hand, training more than six times a week may work against you. Exercising too often can place an undue strain on your muscles, which need time to rest and regenerate between workouts. Unless you are already in peak physical shape, don't push yourself to exercise seven days a week. Too much activity often leads to fatigue, loss of interest in exercise, or worse — injury.

Sometimes hormone fluctuations and other metabolic variables will make you feel stronger than at other times. If you find yourself feeling particularly fit and enthusiastic, try adding an extra set (or more) to each exercise in your workout. Or, you could increase the poundage you are training with. Although it's difficult to offer specific guidelines on increasing poundage, generally speaking you only need to add enough weight to make the exercise challenging, but not too much to prevent you from getting through the entire workout.

Another way you can capitalize on high energy periods is to experiment with training more days of the week than you usually do. If this results in fatigue or stiff and sore muscles, however, you should definitely revert to your regular methods and schedule. It's alright to challenge yourself by making your body work harder, but you've got to 'listen' to your body and take care to avoid injury.

Occasionally, you may have to forgo a week or two of exercise due to illness, travel or time constraints. When this happens, bear in mind that it may take you up to a week to re-attain your former level of conditioning. The safest way to get back in shape after not exercising for a while is to take it gradually, allowing your body and mind to adjust to the demands of working out again.

Pros and Cons of Working Out When You Are Ill

According to John Perretti, owner of the New York gym, Madison Avenue Muscle, 'If you have a cold, your muscles can work. It's perfectly safe to lift weights when you have a cold, since your cardiovascular system isn't really affected. After all, you're working your muscles — you're not building up a sweat inside and you're not hurting your respiratory system. If you have a fever, however, I would advise against training.' Exercising when you have a fever can be dangerous for a number of reasons, so take some time off to recuperate instead of trying to prove your athletic prowess. A few missed days will make little difference in your strength and appearance. You've got the rest of your life to build your body into ideal shape. Regarding minor ailments, such as stomach trouble, earaches, dental work and the like, there's no reason why these conditions should preclude exercise. In fact, working out will probably lessen your discomfort, as increased blood circulation and oxygen levels have an invigorating effect on the body and mind.

'The only thing that stops me from working out is a fever,' claims Beth Rubino. 'I've trained through all kinds of illnesses, and though it's a chore to motivate myself when I'm under par, I get enormous satisfaction from rising above it and exercising in spite of the way I feel. It's very easy to make excuses *not* to work out, so you've got to have the willpower to overcome simple health problems when they arise.'

Notes on Equipment

Although there is a great variety of weight training equipment available today in gyms and in sporting goods stores, there are several points worth considering before joining a gym or purchasing equipment for home workouts. To begin with, there is the question of the relative merits of free weights such as dumb-bells and barbells, and those of the different exercise machines found in most gyms.

Bodybuilders and trainers unanimously agree that free weights afford the muscles a fuller range of resistance and movement (and hence, development) than any exercise machine can provide. When you exercise on a machine, for instance, the balance and control of the weight are maintained by the apparatus. *When lifting free weights, however, it's your muscles that feel the full force of the resistance; it's your muscles which work to balance and control the weight.*

If you happen to be underweight, or your muscles are atrophied, remember that you'll make faster strength and size gains if you use dumb-bells and barbells in lieu of machines. John Perretti, gym owner and bodybuilder, puts it this way: 'The pros and cons of free weights vs machines have been debated for years. Although free weights have their unique benefits, the machinery *is* getting more advanced . . . But if you're interested in making big gains like a 21 in arm, you can't do this without a dumb-bell or barbell. You're never going to get that size from a machine — maybe in the future you will, but right now, no.'

Bear in mind that since you can buy your own set of free weights and exercise at home, you can also save yourself the cost of a health club and gym membership. What you save in money, however, you lose in guidance and camaraderie. Working out in a gym with others, or with a staff trainer, can be immensely helpful to your progress if you decide to become a serious bodybuilder.

Equipment Specifics

As you probably already know, classic progressive resistance exercise equipment includes dumb-bells, a barbell and assorted weight plates that fit interchangeably on both bars. What you may not realize, however, is that old, used weights are just as good as new ones, and buying a used dumb-bell/barbell set could save you a considerable amount of money. Because investing a great deal in exercise equipment can be daunting, why not look in newspaper classified ads for sale notices, or ask in gyms around your town to see if they have any old weights they would like to sell.

Another key piece of equipment for bodybuilders is a *Chinning Bar*. These are excellent for use in vigorous back, shoulder and upper arm workouts. Adjustable chinning bars can be found in most sporting goods stores; they are a relatively inexpensive piece of equipment when bought new. This kind of bar is an adjustable length of metal tubing with rubber tips at each end which are placed across a doorway span and tightened so that the bar will hold your weight. Before you begin exercising on the bar, first check two things:

— Be certain that the bar is lodged tight enough to stay

put. You could injure yourself if you took a fall in the middle of the movement.

— Make sure that the wood of the door jamb is strong enough to hold you and the bar.

Many people who work out like to supplement their weight training programs with aerobic exercises such as jogging for middle distances. One of the most popular fitness trends today involves carrying light *hand weights* (2 to 10 lbs) while running. The weights place extra demands on the cardiovascular system, and some athletes think hand weights help build up the muscle tissue that is somewhat diminished by frequent running workouts. Bruce Nathanson, an allround athlete who has been lifting weights and running marathons for 10 years, says, 'I've used the hand weights to train people who were just coming off smoking 10 to 20 cigarettes a day, and found that they were helpful in getting them to breathe deeper as they ran along . . . and because the weights have built-in grips, they're really easy for people to hold.' Hand weights are available in most sporting goods stores and are extremely inexpensive when you consider the benefits they can provide. For upper body strength and cardiovascular fitness, they're well worth a try.

Regarding equipment for lower body exercises, no guide would be complete without mentioning *Slant Boards*. Useful for doing sit-ups and leg raises at an angle with your feet higher than your hips, slant boards increase the resistance needed to complete the exercise, and so a slant board works your abdominal muscles that much harder.

There are two kinds of slant boards. One is simply a board that has a strap at one end into which you put your feet. To use the board, prop it on a piece of furniture or some other support, and lie head-down to do regular Bent Leg Sit-Ups, etc. The other kind of board is a folding bench which opens up to be a self-supporting, adjustable slant board. Before buying one, however, it's especially important that you test it to see if it's strong enough to hold your weight. Folding slant boards have an added feature that makes them very good buys — they are portable, and fold up into a piece of equipment that you can take anywhere. As with dumb-bell/barbell sets, slant boards are usually just as good used as they are new. Don't let cost stand in the way of challenging workouts — it's perfectly possible to furnish a functional home gym very cheaply.

Acknowledgements

The author would like to thank all those
who contributed to the research and production of
this book. They are: technical consultant Beth
Rubino; Dr. Jairo Rodriguez; John Perretti of Madison
Avenue Muscle; the staff of New York's Natural
Physique Centre; Yvette Diaz; Mary Forsell; Naomi
Black; Michael Montes; Karen Willis and Russel
Lockwood. Photographic models Paul Ludick, Carol
Myers, Nancy Pollak and Michael Reimer deserve
special credit for their hard work and high spirits.

For providing materials and equipment used in
photography, the author would like to thank the
Natural Physique Centre, New York, and Nancy
Pollak Bodywear, also in New York.